ROOT & NOURISH

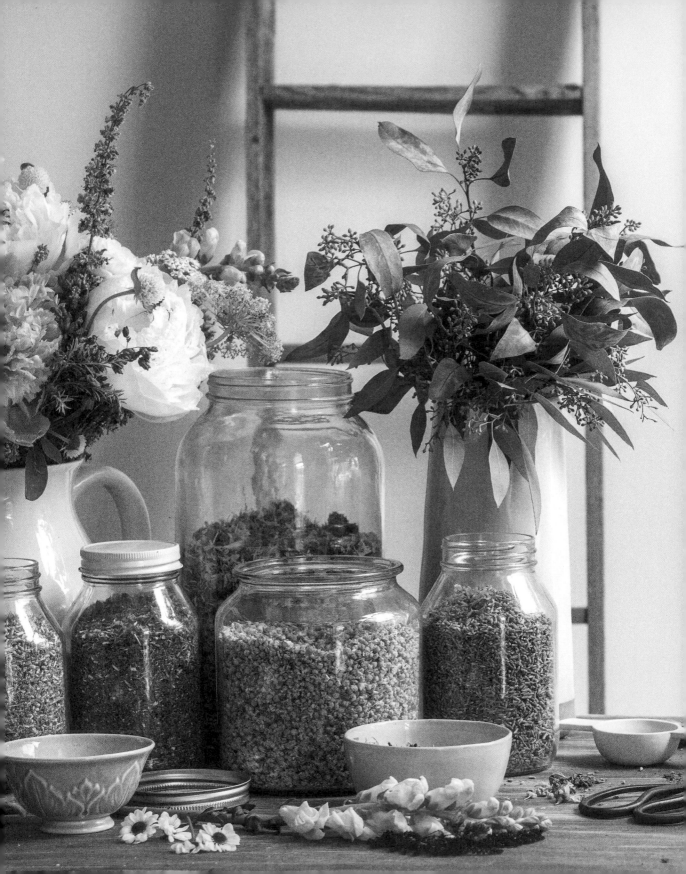

ROOT & NOURISH

AN HERBAL COOKBOOK FOR WOMEN'S WELLNESS

Abbey Rodriguez & Jennifer Kurdyla

TILLER PRESS

NEW YORK   LONDON   TORONTO   SYDNEY   NEW DELHI

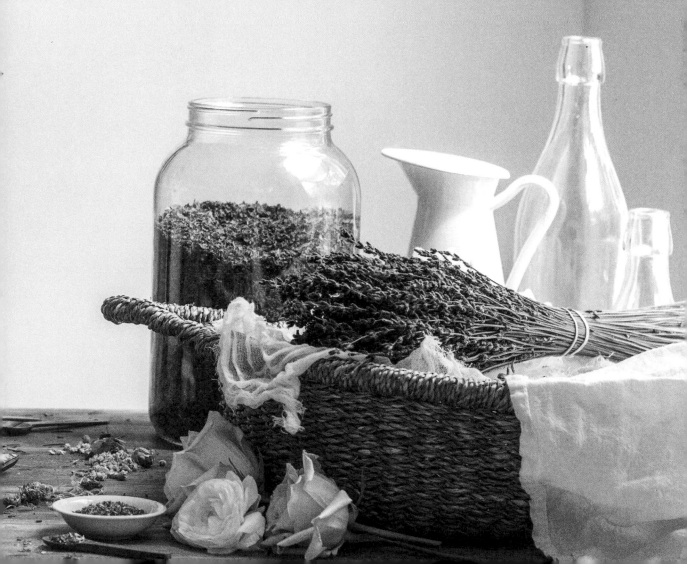

An Imprint of Simon & Schuster, Inc.
1230 Avenue of the Americas
New York, NY 10020

Copyright © 2021 by Abbey Rodriguez and Jennifer Kurdyla

All rights reserved, including the right to reproduce this book or portions
thereof in any form whatsoever. For information, address Simon & Schuster Subsidiary
Rights Department, 1230 Avenue of the Americas, New York, NY 10020.

First Tiller Press hardcover edition April 2021

TILLER PRESS and colophon are trademarks of Simon & Schuster, Inc.

For information about special discounts for bulk purchases, please contact
Simon & Schuster Special Sales at 1-866-506-1949 or business@simonandschuster.com.

The Simon & Schuster Speakers Bureau can bring authors to your live event.
For more information or to book an event, contact the Simon & Schuster Speakers Bureau
at 1-866-248-3049 or visit our website at www.simonspeakers.com.

Interior design by Matthew Ryan
Author photos on page 239 by Matt Rodriguez

Manufactured in the United States of America

10   9   8   7   6   5   4   3   2   1

Library of Congress Cataloging-in-Publication Data has been applied for.

ISBN 978-1-9821-4853-9
ISBN 978-1-9821-4856-0 (ebook)

To our mothers and fathers, in their natural
and human forms—who have given us roots
to keep us nourished, and an insatiable appetite
for eating and living well

I wanted to become a
Wise Woman, grounded
and rooted in the Earth,
listening to its stories
and mediating . . . the old
ancestral and spiritual
wisdom which shows us
how to live in balance in
the world, how to live in
harmony in our communities.

—SHARON BLACKIE, *IF WOMEN ROSE ROOTED*

CONTENTS

SEEDS OF INTEGRATION:
AN HERBAL GUIDE TO HOLISTIC HEALTH 13

How to Use This Book **15**

A Note about Dietary Restrictions **17**

Healing the Earth & Connecting to
the Divine Feminine **18**

KITCHEN APOTHECARY 23

Herbal Actions **26**

THE FIVE PILLARS OF HEALTH 33

TOOLS FOR INTEGRATION 36

HERBAL PANTRY 39

Plant Mylk **43**

Vanilla Extract **44**

Nut & Seed Butters **45**
    Pumpkin Seed Butter **46**
    Almond Butter **47**
    Tahini **47**

Cashew Cream **48**

Soaked Dates **48**

Whipped Coconut Cream
with Marshmallow Root **49**

Plant Parmesan **50**

Umami Spice Blend **50**

Dried Beans **51**

Elderberry Syrup **53**

Herbal Waters **54**
    Warming Digestive Water **54**
    Cleansing Spring Water **54**
    Cooling Summer Water **55**
    Deep Hydration Water **55**
    Anytime Digestive Water **55**

Herbal Balsamic Vinegar **56**

Herbal Cooking Oil **58**

Herbal Vinegar Bitters **59**

PART I: DIGESTION 61

BREAKFAST

Avocado Sauerkraut Toast **66**

Weekday Chia Seed Puddings **67**
    Calming Vanilla & Oats **67**
    Probiotic Elderberry **67**
    Savory Green Goddess **67**
    Double Chocolate Cacao **67**
    Chai This **67**

Essential Banana Bread Muffins **70**

The Rule of Threes for Rooted Digestion **72**

Chamomile Moong Dahl Porridge **73**

Berry Probiotic Açai Bowl **74**

MAINS

Slow & Simple Congee **76**

Coconut Fennel Cashew Curry **77**

Belly Yoga **79**

Probiotic Quinoa Cabbage Stir-Fry **80**

Restorative Kitchari **81**

Wild Dandelion & Mint Pesto **85**

Chunky Fennel, Beet & Chickpea Salsa **86**

Thai Peanut Stir-Fry with Tofu **89**

SWEETS

Baked Apples with Whipped Coconut Cream **90**

Spiced Fig & Berry Compote **93**

Seasonal Eating **94**

Chocolate Almond Butter Oat Bars **96**

TEAS & DRINKS

Cooked Water with Lemon **97**

Ayurvedic CCF Tea **98**

Peppermint Licorice Tea **99**

Chicory Root Cacao **101**

PART II: MENTAL HEALTH 103

BREAKFAST

Spirulina Bliss Smoothie 109

Blueberry, Rose & Walnut Granola 110

Gratitude Reflection 112

Morning-Of Oats 113
   PB&E (Peanut Butter & Elderberry) 113
   Cherry Vanilla 114
   Nuts for Nuts 114
   Mighty Miso Mushroom 115
   Scrambled Plants 115

Vanilla Bean Sweet Potato Banana Pancakes 116

Energizing Sun Salutations 118

MAINS

Ginseng Cilantro Lime Cauliflower Rice 119

Leafy Greens Salad with Walnuts & Berries 120

Heartwarming Vegan Chili 122

Loaded Baked Sweet Potatoes 123

Lemongrass Spring Rolls with Tempeh 124

Cauliflower Pizza with Cashew Cream, Fennel, Arugula & Honey 127

Spaghetti Squash Boats with Basil & Oregano 128

Sourdough for the Soul 130

Spinach Artichoke Cashew Dip 131

Warm Winter Citrus Salad 132

Grounding & Connecting to Plant Energy 135

White Bean Celery Root Soup with Thyme and Rosemary 136

Jackfruit Tacos 137

SWEETS

Super Seed Squares 140

Savory Sage & Flower Tea Biscuits 141

Chai Brown Rice Pudding with Mucuna 142

Alternate Nostril Breathing (Nadi Shodhana Pranayama) 143

Mint Cacao Avocado Pudding 145

Adaptogenic Double Chocolate Brownies 146

Happy Lemon Bars 148

TEAS & DRINKS

Passionflower Mocktail 149

Lemon Balm Lemonade 150

Creamy Chai Latte 152

Cayenne Cacao with Tahini 153

Ayurvedic Psychology (Sattva, Rajas, & Tamas) 154

Lavender, Chamomile & Rose Tea 157

Gentle Yoga for Relaxation 158

Herbal Lullaby Tea 159

PART III: FEMALE REPRODUCTIVE HORMONAL HEALTH 161

BREAKFAST

Balanced Beauty Bowl with Schisandra 167

PMS Smoothie 168

Apple Oat Smoothie Bowl 169

Grain-Free Seed Granola, Four Ways 170

Moon Glow—Lunar Cycles & Rituals to Connect to the Divine Feminine 176

MAINS

Avocado Womb Bowl 179

Shakshuka with Plant-Based Egg 180

Crunchy Seaweed Wrap 182

White Bean Beet Hummus 184

Supported Goddess Pose (Supta Baddha Konasana) 185

Golden Cream of Beet Soup 186

Creamy Broccoli Soup 188

Roasted Brussels Sprouts, Sweet Potato & Tempeh Bowl with Fenugreek Dressing 189

Mushroom Risotto with Spinach, Peas & Nettles 193

SWEETS

Bliss Bites 195
  Matcha Bites 195
  Dark Chocolate Fig Oatmeal Bites 197
  Cookie Dough Bites 197
  Pumpkin Seed Cacao Bites 198
  Moon Glow Bites 199
  Double Chocolate Bliss Bites 200

Curate Your Own Wellness Altar 201

Peanut Butter Licorice Fudge 204

Adaptogenic Chocolate Chip Cookies 207

Tahini Truffles 208

TEAS & DRINKS

Spicy Turmeric Latte 209

Cycle Support Teas 210
  Milk Thistle & Nettle 210
  Red Raspberry Leaf & Hibiscus 210

Garden Goddess Tonic 213

Rose Cacao 214

Self-Love Self-Massage (Abhyanga) 215

Pink Moon Mylk 217

Ojas Mylk 218

Your Ojas is Glowing 219

ROOT & NOURISH—DAILY RITUALS 220

FURTHER STUDY 223

HERBAL SUPPLIERS 224

ACKNOWLEDGMENTS 225

INDEX 228

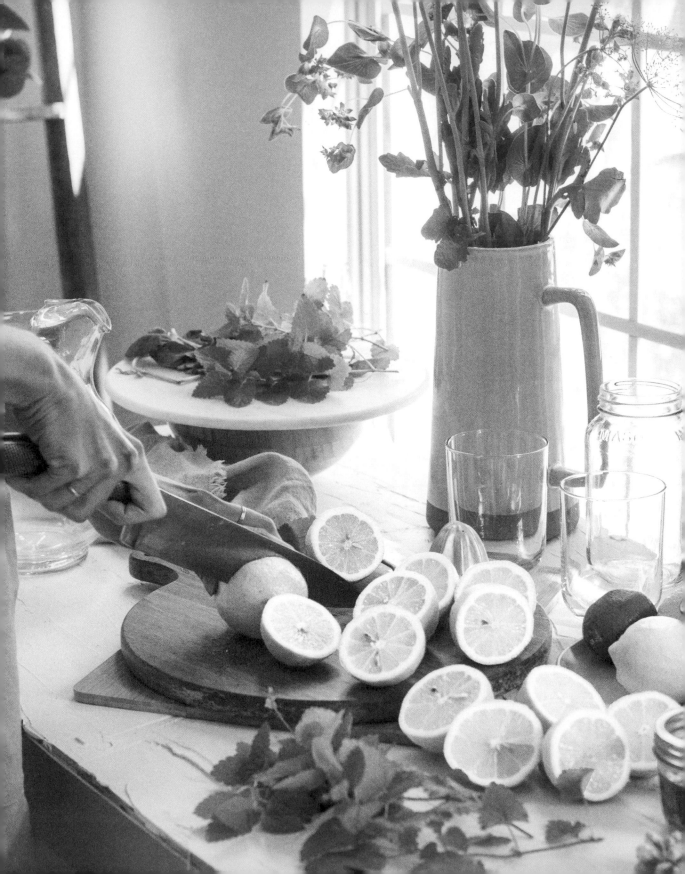

SEEDS OF INTEGRATION
AN HERBAL GUIDE TO HOLISTIC HEALTH

When you think about what healthy means to you, what comes to mind? Perhaps it's glowing skin, lush hair, or the absence of disease—one of the chronic lifestyle diseases common in our society, such as diabetes or hypertension, or an acute illness that keeps you away for a few days from the activities and people you love. Health can be those things, but it's also much, much more. Health is not merely something that appears on the outside, in the form of social media posts or the results of a blood test. Rather, it's an integrated and ever-evolving balancing act involving all the many systems of your body, the environment, and the state of your mind, emotions, and spirit.

At least, that is the perspective of health from which we come to you in this book. In our years as humans on the earth, we have confronted a range of health concerns—chronic and acute, personally and professionally—and we have run through the gamut of conventional medical resources in our attempts to find cures for them. Western medicine has been instrumental in providing useful diagnoses and treatments to that end, yet holistic practices have been the most sustainable, nourishing, and effective ways to restore and maintain health in its broadest meaning. Through both Western herbalism and Ayurveda, we've discovered not cures, but healing.

The word "healing" has its roots in the Dutch and German words for "whole," an idea that pervades and connects these two modalities at the core of *Root & Nourish*. (Hence the use of the term "holistic" to describe these and other wellness systems, like Traditional Chinese Medicine.) While they stem from different parts of the world, and each has its own incredibly rich lineage, Western herbalism and Ayurveda share the idea that nature alone has the power to bring us into a state of health—and keep us there. Since we are part of nature, that power also resides in us, but only when we see ourselves as whole, integrated beings. When we remember that we are part of the vast universe of nature's wholeness, connected to each other and all living things, and sync back into the rhythms, instincts, and changes of Earth, we can discover healing from the inside out.

Holistic healing won't happen without our participation: In other words, we need to be mindful about putting into (and onto) our bodies things that are wholesome and nourishing if we expect to get wholeness and nourishment out of them. Western herbalism and Ayurveda both turn to plants for those high-quality inputs, with an extensive pharmacopoeia of plant-based medicines—teas, tinctures, decoctions, formulas, and topical products that draw on the myriad innate qualities of different plants (which we'll explore throughout this book, so get excited) to bring us back to our state of nature. You see, plants are a mirror of our own energetics, nutrients, and sense of integration, so if we've lost some of that due to illness, we can turn to plants to replenish those qualities in us.

Ask any holistic practitioner, however, and they'll tell you that herbal medicines are never the first line of defense. Medicines take the power of plants and concentrate them into a form that will work more quickly and specifically (in most cases), and that's great if we're in some kind of health crisis. (That's not to say herbal medicine is a substitute for Western medicine—they can, and should, support each other. Herbs work much more slowly and systemically than most Western protocols, which is why if you break your arm or are having a heart attack, we wouldn't try to treat that with herbs. Holistic and conventional medicine need each other to provide balanced healthcare—a kind of wholeness in and of itself.)

But what if we're not in a health crisis, but just feeling a little off? And what if we're feeling well—how do we prevent a health crisis from happening?

Here's where herbs—and this book—come into the picture. We can use herbs (and spices)—the most potent form of plants' energy—to engage with long-term and preventive healing in the form of food. By taking wholesome plants into our bodies every day, multiple times a day, we are essentially microdosing on plant medicine, and in doing so building up stores of immunity, repairing minor damage at a cellular level, efficiently eliminating waste, and keeping all parts of us communicating with each other and working together. (This applies if you don't follow a plant-based diet—animals eat plants, so the quality of their food matters to you, too.) Eating whole plant foods rather than taking an isolated, processed drug form of even those same nutrients will always provide a more integrated healing experience. Consider the wisdom of an Ayurvedic proverb: "When diet is wrong, medicine is of no use. When diet is correct, medicine is of no need."

The idea of treating food as medicine is not one that came to us naturally on our health journey. Our society attaches confusing morality to food in its messaging—which foods are "clean" and which are "toxic," how much and how often we should eat, and other rules and judgments. By relying solely on these external messages circulating in the media for guidance on how and what to eat, ranging from fad diets to conflicting scientific studies, we've become disconnected from the internal wisdom of our bodies. We've collectively lost our ability to eat well, the most fundamental ritual any of us could do in service to our present and future health. It's no wonder that so many of us have become accustomed to living with a wide array of digestive, mental health, and hormonal imbalances. The root cause of our collective dis-ease is inside of us and tied to what and how we're feeding ourselves.

If we're looking to be more mindful in what we consume for the purposes of whole-body healing, we need a wider definition of "food." There's the stuff we grow, harvest, cook with, and consume—the kind of food we'll talk about mostly in this book. But our environment, relationships, sensory experiences, and all the external stimuli we come into contact with are kinds of food, too. Those parts of our diet have an enormous effect not only on how we feel physically, but mentally, emotionally, and spiritually—just like regular food. We can apply the same priorities of wholeness and nourishment we use to determine how we fill our plate to determining how we fill these other parts of our lives, if we want to create a truly holistic lifestyle.

The good news about this is that the solution to that dis-ease is also inside you. Through the recipes and other self-care practices we've compiled in *Root & Nourish*, you'll have all you need to remember your innate knowledge of wholeness and healing, so you can be the most rooted and nourished version of yourself inside and out.

HOW TO USE THIS BOOK

These recipes were designed with specific intentions to achieve a desired effect based on the known properties of the ingredients, but there is no one-size-fits-all recipe for health. That mentality is actually quite the opposite of the personalized health care offered by Western herbalism and Ayurvedic traditions. As such, if there are ingredients that don't serve you for any reason, by all means substitute them with something you like better or can access. Pay attention to your intuition and the herbs that call to you with their color, fragrance, and taste.

We've also tried to keep our techniques and tools simple, so cooks with any level of experience can enjoy these recipes. With that in mind, there is no obligation to follow our instructions or process perfectly. If you have another method of cooking rice, like your sweet potatoes sliced instead of cubed, or don't have a citrus press, you can still make lemonade (real and metaphorical). We encourage you to experiment, tweak, and use these recipes as templates for developing your own culinary self-care skills.

There are two ways you might approach the start of your herbal cooking journey in this book. First, consider the three sections into which we have divided the recipes. Part I focuses on digestion, where optimal health begins and ends. If you've ever been to a holistic practitioner, they've probably asked you about your poop in a way that might have been new to you, and even a little strange, at the time. But poop, and all that goes into it, is a key indicator of our ability to digest our food and, by extension, everything else our senses take in. Part I offers foods that support the full spectrum of upset bellies to lead you toward your own optimal digestive patterns. No matter what you're dealing with individually, the general principle here is to give the digestive system a rest from the nonstop intake of foods, information, emotions, people, and energies that may be throwing you off course. Simple, well cooked, and mildly spiced foods come to the rescue here. Once things are back in order, you might find you need to further stimulate or calm the GI tract with specific herbs and foods, including those that feed the microbiome and encourage healthy elimination.

Part II goes into the mind—which doesn't only mean your brain. Achieving balanced mental health has just as much to do with your gut as it does the organ inside your skull. Our digestive system houses the body's largest concentration of serotonin, a hormone that sends signals of happiness throughout the system (among other things). The gut has its own way of communicating, called the enteric nervous system, that can bypass the central nervous system entirely to send out those signals of happiness, as well as other feelings you might know as "gut feelings." The foods we use to nourish our mental health—whether we're living with stress (and all that implies), anxiety, depression, insomnia, mood imbalances, and/or low energy—can bring balance to those receptors in the gut as well as throughout the central nervous system. The other big nutrient that can't be itemized on a nutrition label is pleasure. When we eat food that makes us happy, with people and in places that make us happy, too, our bodies digest that food better and then function and feel better. You'll therefore find a number of recipes in this section meant to indulge in and share, so you're feeding yourself a daily dose of joy.

Part III takes us to our reproductive system, where we can examine more long-term effects of proper (or improper) nourishment. You see, the body is very smart, and it evolved to prioritize survival—a good thing! What this means, though, is that it will always allocate more resources to the systems and chemicals (i.e., hormones) that will keep us out of danger—ones that put us in a state of alertness, guardedness, and stress so we can fight or flee from danger. Back in the day, when danger looked like bears wandering into our cavepeople camps, that stress response (governed by the sympathetic nervous system) would turn on when needed, we'd shake it off (literally), and go back to our lives. In our current world, though, those triggers are going off all the time, leaving us perpetually tense and on edge—hence the situation we address in Part II.

When the body is worried about bears, it can't also be taking care of things like digestion and elimination, immunity, cell repair and communication, or reproduction—the latter being what we'll focus on in Part III. (After all, if you're being chased by a bear, being able to conceive a child is not really a priority.) It's this imbalance of stimulating stress hormones and nourishing reproductive hormones that can be behind our reproductive concerns, as well as digestive and mental health concerns. See how it's all connected?

While the specifics of all the possible reproductive concerns women may have (from menstruation through fertility, conception, pregnancy, and birth, to menopause and beyond) are outside the scope of this book, we do offer ways to support the reproductive tissues and hormones with powerful plant medicine. Considering the integrated reproductive systems of plants—how tiny seeds develop into strong and deep roots, graceful stems, and beautiful flowers and fruits—consuming them in their whole-food form is in and of itself a nourishing way to access the generative energy of our bodies. The ingredients we've chosen for the recipes in Part III borrow from indigenous practices from around the world, including adaptogens, tonics, and plants with aphrodisiac properties that specifically target our reproductive system.

If you're not sure which part of this book best serves you—perhaps you have a number of conditions, or you don't have a specific diagnosis but are just looking to feel better in your day-to-day—don't stress (and we mean that!). Follow your intuition and cravings for whatever recipes jump out at you. As described above, all the sections in this book support each other, so you can start anywhere you like and move through the recipes in any order. Cravings can also be important guides for what your body needs from a nutritional standpoint, so enjoying what you're in the mood for on any given day can be an important and beneficial way to practice self-awareness and mindful eating. Feeding those cravings with wild foods and herbs will further allow us to live in closer harmony with the cycles and rhythms of the natural world. By embracing this holistic view, you'll be stepping away from the reductionist symptom- and disease-based definition of health, and into an entire way of living that feeds more than just your body.

Indeed, working holistically with herbs doesn't have to stop at your plate. Because of all the ways that we can be nourished beyond food, it's important to incorporate a holistic mind-set into your entire lifestyle as part of a full-body, full-spirit journey to wellness. To that end, throughout the book you'll find special "Rooted Living" sections, which spotlight certain Ayurvedic and yogic practices to infuse your entire day with healing energy. If you're new to yoga, it's best to consult with a trained teacher before beginning a full practice, but the offerings here are gentle enough for anyone with any level of experience. Try a few or try them all, see which fit into your schedule, and notice how they affect your feelings around what and how you eat. You may even discover that self-care feeds emotional or stress-based food cravings, helping you make better decisions for your long-term health.

All the recipes and suggestions in this book are intended for anyone to use safely and in moderation, not for the purposes of diagnosing or treating illness. We cannot emphasize enough that herbs have powerful and unique effects on each of us. If you have preexisting conditions, are taking medications, or would simply like

more targeted guidance on herbal medicine, please consult a healthcare provider or herbal practitioner. They will be able to advise you on the best practices to meet your needs.

A NOTE ABOUT DIETARY RESTRICTIONS

We advocate for plant-based, gluten-free foods for several reasons, none of which are absolute and right for everyone. There is an abundance of data supporting the health benefits of a plant-based diet. By respecting animal life, we are also contributing to the overall health of the environment, both ecological and spiritual.

When it comes to gluten, there are real reasons to avoid it entirely—such as when there is a diagnosed allergy. Sensitivities, however, are another thing, at least from the holistic perspective. Our society's general overconsumption of gluten is behind some people's sensitivities, and avoiding gluten (and other inflammatory foods) is often beneficial— for a short time. When we avoid food groups altogether over an extended period, though, those sensitivities can get exacerbated. We are not suggesting you deliberately eat anything that causes you pain. But you may find that as you work on healing your gut (and by extension, your mind and hormones), you can tolerate more gluten without discomfort. If you are already fine eating gluten, then you should not feel the need to eliminate it, and are welcome to replace any of the gluten-free grains or products called for in the recipes with others of your choice.

Additionally of note is our use of honey in select recipes. Honey is the source of much debate among the plant-based community: It is an "animal product," yet it is essential to the flourishing of many edible plants at the core of a vegan diet. Widespread honeybee deaths are also an increasing problem for the global ecosystems. We support the use of honey because of its overall sustainability when compared to other processed vegan sweeteners (such as agave nectar and brown rice syrup), and for its health benefits, especially when consumed raw and sourced locally. Honey's antimicrobial, immune-boosting, and astringent properties also make it a potent medicine in herbal traditions, and you may view it as such when consuming it. But again, if honey is not part of your diet, you're welcome to substitute it; however, you may find that alternative sweeteners alter the consistency and flavor of the finished dish.

Note that honey should never be cooked, as doing so breaks down its live enzymes so they are indigestible, making a harmful substance known in Ayurveda as *āma*. If you're using honey to sweeten tea, simply allow the tea to cool for a few minutes until it's a temperature you'd drink it at, or until you can hold your pinky finger in the liquid for 10 seconds, and then add the honey.

HEALING THE EARTH & CONNECTING TO THE DIVINE FEMININE

The benefits of food extends far beyond what it does for us nutritionally. It is a catalyst for connection, tradition, and the many beautiful parts of life that we hold in highest value—which for us humans includes the planet we live on. Numerous scientific studies show our need for connection to the natural world in order to maintain an optimal state of well-being, but this knowledge has been part of indigenous traditions for centuries. Today, our coexistence with nature has decreased, and in many ways, we have lost touch with how to be a part of the natural world—how to be fully present in our bodies and senses and embrace the cycles of the seasons.

Herbalism is intrinsically in tune with nature. Because it operates within the context of our collective ecological and evolutionary legacy with the plant queendom, it has been described as "ecological healing." Its practices offer particular and essential expressions of cooperating with nature and can help us remember our intuitive connection to plants. The more we know about the plants we live among, the more we will be inclined to respect them with all of our daily routines—how and what we eat in terms of foods; our consumption of plastics and other packaging; our food and other waste; chemical additives in our clothing, beauty, hygiene, and cleaning products; our transportation, and more. You wouldn't serve your mother a big mug of gasoline, so why would you do the same to your mother the Earth, who takes care of all living beings equally and completely and asks for nothing in return?

Respecting the Earth also requires moderation, something that our society doesn't value. We see ads for herbal products (any product, really), and think more of it must be better. The truth is, enough is the best amount of any medicine, plant or otherwise, and when we're in sync with our bodies' messages we will know when we've had enough and stop there. Consider this as you are cooking with herbs. Notice that the quantities in the recipes tend to be small— fractions of teaspoons for an entire dish. You can

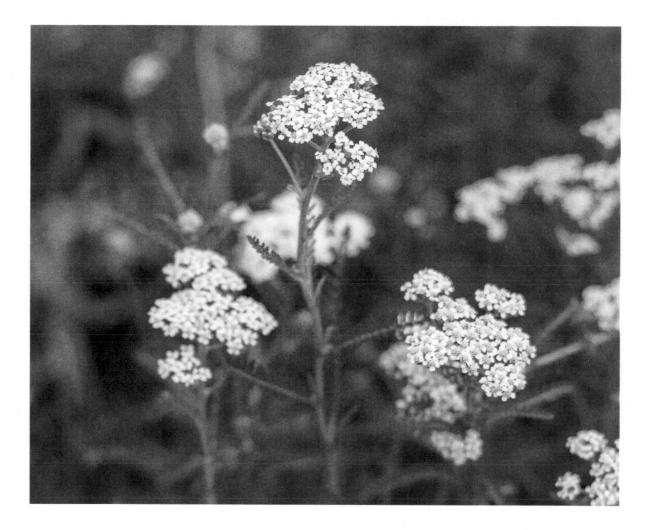

always add more if needed, but it's a lot harder to take out ingredients! By only taking what we need, no more and no less, we're ensuring there is enough medicine on the planet for everyone who needs it, today and in the future. To that end, we have purposefully selected ingredients that are not on the at-risk list of herbs curated by United Plant Savers, so that herbalism does not become an additional strain on our natural resources. You can find out more about sustainable herbalism in our Further Study section on page 223.

Getting in tune with nature might sound a bit antiquated to you—and it is. Part of the process of reconnecting to ourselves involves stripping away the veils of convenience, speed, and instant gratification that defines our culture. It is the way of ancient and living indigenous cultures, who thrived for centuries without energy drinks or iPhones. These are the cultures whose innate connections to the earth are at the root of modern herbal practices, which we are honored to share with you in these pages to the best of our ability.

We hope to continue the line of wise women who have served as ambassadors of nature and thank you for taking on the responsibility of joining these traditions with intentionality and enthusiasm as well.

As women, we also have a special role to play in our individual and collective realignment with nature. Getting closer to the earth as a means of rejuvenating health helped us personally discover a deeper connection to Mother Earth and our own unique experience of our female bodies, in states of disease and wellness alike. It's alarming to consider that the prevalence of digestive, mental, and hormonal health concerns we discuss in this book is much greater in women than men. At the same time, the Earth is also hurting, ravaged by the effects of climate change, pollution, and industrial agriculture practices that feed our Mother with the wrong kind of nutrition. Thus, in choosing what and how we eat with greater intention and clarity, we are able to nurture our female selves as much as the Earth's, our ultimate source of health. As Sharon Blackie writes in *If Women Rose Rooted*: "If women remember that once upon a time we sang with the seals and flew with the wings of swans, that we forged our own paths through the dark forest while creating a community of its many inhabitants, then we will rise up rooted, like trees. And if we rise up rooted, like trees . . . well then, women might indeed save not only ourselves, but the world."

This healing power applies regardless of our gender identity; all people possess both feminine and masculine energy (what the Chinese Medicine system calls *yin* and *yang*), and harnessing more of the feminine energy—with its grounding, nurturing, compassionate, and slow qualities— would help us all resist the larger social ills of greed, burnout, and judgment that are at the root of so much dis-ease. If we want to help our bodies' creative capacities function optimally— through reproduction as well as professional and creative "offspring"—we cannot block the creative capacity of the Earth; we must treat its resources as we do our own, with respect and generosity.

While our own experiences and expertise are behind the combination of Western herbalism and Ayurveda in this book, the two systems stem from the same roots of indigenous practices not necessarily our own. Our intention is to offer you the most relevant teachings from Western and Eastern traditions. They may use different languages (literal and figurative) to describe the properties of plants, or even rely on different plants themselves based on where they're grown natively, but the space where they overlap in the Venn diagram of herbalism is larger than where they are separate. This symbiosis of two types of herbalism is a kind of holistic practice in and of itself, and we acknowledge that it will not allow for a complete understanding of either system. We hope to offer a fair and accurate representation of certain concepts and tools from these systems to the best of our knowledge. And we encourage you to join us on a path of study that will likely continue beyond this lifetime.

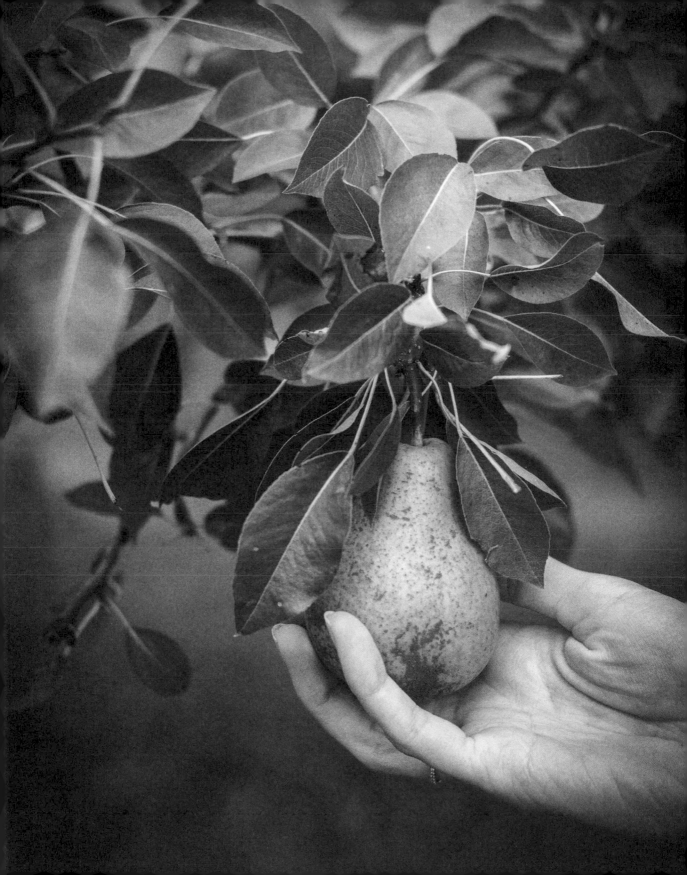

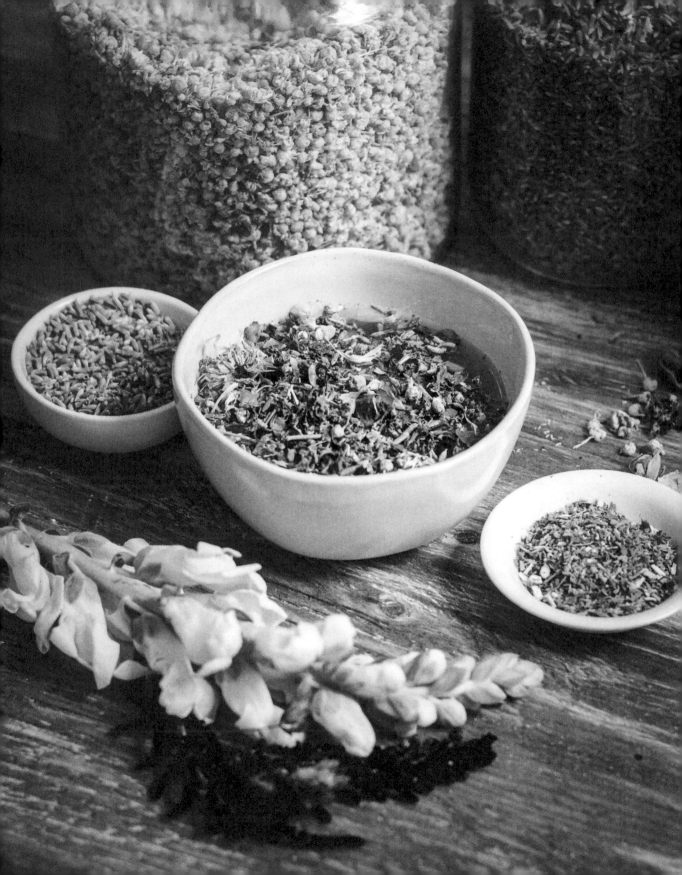

KITCHEN APOTHECARY

The complete catalog of herbal medicine spans many books, which is one reason why herbalism can seem overwhelming to people at first. Knowing which herbs to buy, what they do, and how to consume them may not seem intuitive, but we're here to reassure you that the process of building an herbal apothecary in your own home can be simple, fun, and beautiful. By welcoming herbs, even if it's just a single jar of chamomile or a vase of roses, into your home—your body and the place where you live—you're communing with our shared home, the earth, and inviting the kind of energy that will restore balance in both micro and macro ways.

The following pages include a list of all of the herbs we use in this book. You may recognize many of the ingredients, while others might be newer to you, or less available depending on where you live.

Before you go out and buy them all, we encourage you to take time working through the recipes to know which ones you'll be using more or less often. (See page 224 for trusted sources of herbs.) As they are superfoods, you can get a lot of medicine from a small quantity of herbs but buying in bulk might help you save time and money once you find your herb soul mate(s). Growing your own herbs is a fantastic idea if you can. You don't need a farm or even a backyard to engage with plants—a simple pot of basil (regular or Holy) in an apartment windowsill can serve as a mighty lifeline to Mother Nature. We've highlighted some of our favorite, most-often used herbs throughout the book in the "Nourishing Herbs" boxes. Unless otherwise noted, all the herbs below can be used in their dried and/or powdered form. The recipes will indicate any special forms.

ASHWAGANDHA (*WITHANIA SOMNIFERA*)	powder
ASIAN GINSENG (*PANAX GINSENG*)	powder
BASIL (*OCIMUM BASILICUM*)	fresh and dried
BLACK PEPPER (*PIPER NIGRUM*)	whole peppercorns and ground
CALENDULA (*CALENDULA OFFICINALIS*)	fresh and dried flowers
CARDAMOM (*ELETTARIA CARDAMOMUM*)	whole green pods and ground
CAYENNE (*CAPSICUM FRUTESCENS/ANNUUM*)	powder
CHAMOMILE (*MATRICARIA CHAMOMILLA*)	dried flowers
CHICORY ROOT (*CICHORIUM INTYBUS*)	dried
CILANTRO (*CORIANDRUM SATIVUM*)	fresh (as Coriander, whole seeds and ground)
CINNAMON (*CINNAMOMUN VERUM*)	sticks and ground
CLOVE (*SYZYGIUM AROMATICUM*)	whole and ground
CUMIN (*CUMINUM CYMINUM*)	whole seeds and ground
DANDELION (*TARAXACUM OFFICINALE*)	fresh greens and dried root
ELDERBERRY (*SAMBUCUS NIGRA SUBSP. CANADENSIS*)	dried
FENNEL (*FOENICULUM VULGARE*)	fresh and whole seeds
GARLIC (*ALLIUM SATIVUM*)	fresh and ground
GINGER (*ZINGIBER OFFICINALE*)	fresh and ground
HIBISCUS (*HIBISCUS SABDARIFFA*)	dried flowers and powder
HING (*FERULA ASSA-FOETIDA*)	powder
LAVENDER (*LAVANDULA ANGUSTIFOLIA*)	dried culinary-grade flowers
LEMON BALM (*MELISSA OFFICINALIS*)	fresh
LEMONGRASS (*CYMBOPOGON CITRATUS*)	fresh
LICORICE ROOT (*GLYCYRRHIZA GLABRA*)	whole root and powder
MACA (*LEPIDIUM MEYENII*)	gelatinized powder
MARSHMALLOW ROOT (*ALTHAEA*)	dried
MATCHA (*CAMELLIA SINENSIS*)	powder
MUCUNA (*MUCUNA PRURIENS*)	powder

NETTLES (*URTICA DIOICA*)	dried
NUTMEG (*MYRISTICA FRAGRANS*)	ground
OATSTRAW (*AVENA SATIVA*)	dried
PARSLEY (*PETROSELINUM CRISPUM*)	fresh and dried
PASSIONFLOWER (*PASSIFLORA*)	dried
PEPPERMINT (*MENTHA PIPERITA*)	fresh and dried
PSYLLIUM (*PLANTAGO PSYLLIUM*)	husk powder
RED RASPBERRY LEAF (*RUBUS IDAEUS*)	dried
REISHI (*GANODERMA LUCIDUM*)	powder
ROSE (*ROSA DAMASCENA*)	culinary-grade dried rose petals and powder
SAGE (*SALVIA OFFICINALIS*)	fresh and dried
SEEDS	raw, untoasted, unsalted, hulled
CHIA SEEDS (*SALVIA HISPANICA*)	
FLAXSEEDS (*LINUM USITATISSIMUM*)	
PUMPKIN SEEDS (*CUCURBITA PEPO*)	
SESAME SEEDS (*SESAMUM INDICUM*)	
SUNFLOWER SEEDS (*HELIANTHUS ANNUUS*)	
SHATAVARI (*ASPARAGUS RACEMOSUS*)	powder
SHIITAKE (*LENTINULA EDODES*)	dried mushroom and powder
SKULLCAP (*SCUTELLARIA*)	dried
SPIRULINA (*ARTHROSPIRA*)	powder
THYME (*THYMUS VULGARIS*)	fresh and dried
TULSI (*OCIMUM TENUIFLORUM*)	dried
TURMERIC (*CURCUMA LONGA*)	ground
YARROW (*ACHILLEA MILLEFOLIUM*)	dried

HERBAL ACTIONS

We can use herbs as medicine because their inherent properties, known as herbal actions, have an affinity with certain systems of the human body. Take a moment to let that soak in—how miraculous is it that plants and our bodies are hard-wired to work with each other? This symbiosis is exactly what we mean when we talk about a holistic approach to health—when we work with plants, we're basically realigning our bodies with themselves, rather than using an external agent (like a drug) to force change, suppress, or control.

Herbal actions help to describe the categories of herbs, so that when we're looking for certain results, we know which herbs to turn to first. However, as you'll see from the list below, many herbs fall into multiple categories. Unlike the kind of support you'd find in a vitamin capsule, which is often made of an isolated compound, consuming the whole herb means that you're getting multiple benefits, and in the form nature intended it to be consumed for maximum compatibility with your body. Turmeric is one common example of how this works. Many people take curcumin capsules, which is the main compound in turmeric root and can be sold at higher concentrations than you'd be able to consume from just eating turmeric (a great line for marketers to get you to buy more pills). However, whole turmeric root has many other compounds in it that allow for that curcumin to be absorbed fully by your system. Sprinkling some turmeric on your food or making our Spicy Turmeric Latte (page 209), is therefore the more holistic—and healing—way to get all the herbal benefits of this plant—as an alterative, anti-inflammatory, antioxidant, astringent, and multi-system tonic.

In each section of the book we will highlight which groups of herbal actions and individual herbs are being called upon most in the recipes. Feel free to refer here to refresh your memory on what the actions do. Note that the list of herbal actions below is not exhaustive, but highlights those relevant to these recipes. As you experiment with your kitchen apothecary, take note of which actions you're leaning into most often, and what their effects on your system are at different points along your journey. Over time, you'll start to build a relationship with certain herbs, so that your choices for cooking are guided by intuition, not merely looking up references in a book.

ADAPTOGENIC

Herbs that support and nourish the adrenals (where stress hormones are produced) and increase resilience to stressors in a nonspecific way.

+ Ashwagandha
+ Asian ginseng
+ Licorice root
+ Maca
+ Mucuna

+ Reishi
+ Schisandra
+ Shatavari
+ Shiitake
+ Tulsi

ALTERATIVE

Herbs that purify the blood, cleanse lymph, and increase the function of elimination channels through the liver, kidneys, skin, and lungs.

+ Calendula
+ Cilantro
+ Dandelion root

+ Elderberry
+ Tulsi
+ Turmeric

ANTI-INFLAMMATORY

Herbs that support the reduction of inflammation in the body and disrupt the prostaglandin process. Prostaglandins are lipids (fats) made at places where tissue damage or inflammation occurs. Anti-inflammatory herbs disrupt that process so inflammation is decreased.

+ Ashwagandha
+ Calendula
+ Chamomile
+ Cilantro
+ Cumin
+ Elderberry
+ Fennel
+ Fenugreek
+ Flaxseed
+ Licorice root
+ Nettle
+ Nutmeg
+ Peppermint
+ Reishi
+ Tulsi
+ Turmeric
+ Yarrow

ANTIMICROBIAL

Herbs that support the body in destroying pathogenic microorganisms.

+ Calendula
+ Cayenne
+ Chamomile
+ Cinnamon
+ Cloves
+ Garlic
+ Lemon balm
+ Tulsi

ANTIOXIDANT

Herbs that reduce the circulation of free radicals, the harmful by-products of the body's natural detoxification process that cause damage to cells, proteins, and DNA.

+ Black pepper
+ Cayenne
+ Cinnamon
+ Clove
+ Elderberry
+ Oatstraw
+ Reishi
+ Sage
+ Spirulina
+ Tulsi
+ Turmeric

ANTISPASMODIC

Herbs that ease cramps and reduce the intensity of muscle spasms.

+ Basil
+ Calendula
+ Cayenne
+ Chamomile
+ Cumin
+ Elderberry
+ Garlic
+ Hing
+ Lavender
+ Lemon balm
+ Licorice root
+ Nutmeg
+ Oatstraw
+ Passionflower
+ Peppermint
+ Rose
+ Skullcap
+ Yarrow

APERIENT

Herbs that work as a gentle laxative, to stimulate the digestive system and aid the work of the liver.

+ Chicory root
+ Elderberry
+ Flaxseed
+ Psyllium

APHRODISIAC

Herbs that nourish the nervous, cardiovascular, and reproductive systems on both physical and energetic levels; tonify the body and support balanced function; and enhance sexual desire (libido) and performance.

+ Ashwagandha
+ Asian ginseng
+ Fenugreek
+ Ginger
+ Hibiscus
+ Maca
+ Mucuna
+ Oatstraw
+ Rose
+ Shatavari

ASTRINGENT

Herbs that have a binding effect on mucus membranes, skin, and other tissues to tone and tighten.

+ Ashwagandha
+ Cinnamon
+ Hibiscus
+ Lemongrass
+ Red raspberry leaf
+ Sage
+ Schisandra
+ Thyme
+ Turmeric
+ Yarrow

BITTER

Herbs that act as stimulant tonics for the digestive system through a reflex to their bitter taste via the taste buds.

+ Chamomile
+ Chicory root
+ Dandelion root

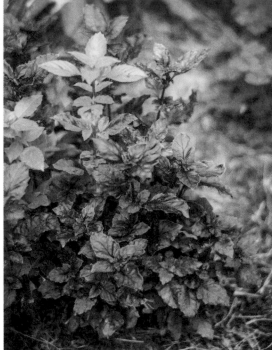

CARMINATIVE

Herbs that are rich in volatile oils, which reduce gas, relax the stomach, and stimulate peristalsis (downward movement) of the digestive system.

+ Basil
+ Black pepper
+ Cardamom
+ Cayenne
+ Chamomile
+ Cilantro
+ Cinnamon
+ Cloves
+ Cumin
+ Elderberry
+ Fennel
+ Fenugreek
+ Garlic
+ Ginger
+ Hing
+ Lavender
+ Lemon balm
+ Nutmeg
+ Parsley
+ Peppermint
+ Tulsi

DEMULCENT

Herbs rich in mucilage, which soothes and protects irritated or inflamed internal tissue.

+ Chia seed
+ Fenugreek
+ Flaxseed
+ Licorice root
+ Marshmallow root
+ Oatstraw
+ Psyllium
+ Tulsi

EMMENAGOGUE

Herbs that tone and stimulate the female reproductive system.

+ Calendula
+ Cilantro
+ Cumin
+ Fenugreek
+ Hibiscus
+ Lavender
+ Lemongrass
+ Maca
+ Nettle
+ Peppermint
+ Red raspberry leaf
+ Rose
+ Sage
+ Yarrow

HEPATIC

Herbs that strengthen and protect the liver.

+ Chicory root
+ Dandelion
+ Licorice root
+ Reishi

LAXATIVE

Herbs that help promote elimination of bowels.

+ Chicory root
+ Ginger
+ Licorice root
+ Psyllium

NERVINE

Herbs that restore and strengthen the nervous system.

Relaxants

+ Chamomile
+ Lavender
+ Lemon balm
+ Lemongrass
+ Mucuna
+ Oatstraw
+ Passionflower
+ Peppermint
+ Rose
+ Skullcap
+ Tulsi

PHYTOESTROGENIC

Herbs containing any of a diverse group of compounds that can bind to estrogen-receptor sites and elicit an estrogenic effect; used for female reproductive disorders.

+ Calendula
+ Fennel
+ Flaxseed
+ Licorice root
+ Maca
+ Pumpkin seeds
+ Sage
+ Sesame seeds
+ Sunflower seeds

SEDATIVE

Herbs that reduce stress, calm the nervous system, and calm feelings of overwhelm; many sedative herbs can be taken before bed to promote restful sleep.

+ Ashwagandha
+ Asian ginseng
+ Chamomile
+ Lavender
+ Lemon balm
+ Passionflower
+ Skullcap

TONICS

Herbs that nourish, tone, balance, and restore natural function, vitality, and flexibility to tissues and/or organs.

ADRENAL TONICS:

+ Ashwagandha
+ Licorice root
+ Asian ginseng

DIGESTIVE TONICS:

+ Chicory root
+ Turmeric
+ Dandelion

IMMUNE TONICS:

+ Reishi
+ Tulsi
+ Shiitake
+ Turmeric

LIVER TONICS:

+ Licorice root
+ Turmeric
+ Nettle

NERVOUS SYSTEM TONICS:

+ Ashwagandha
+ Oatstraw
+ Fenugreek
+ Rose
+ Mucuna
+ Skullcap

UTERINE TONICS:

+ Fenugreek
+ Red raspberry leaf
+ Nettle
+ Rose

VULNERARY

Herbs that are wound-healers (internal and external use).

+ Calendula
+ Oatstraw
+ Chamomile
+ Yarrow

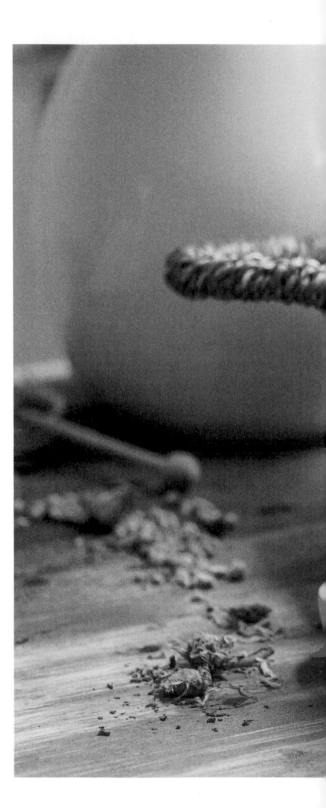

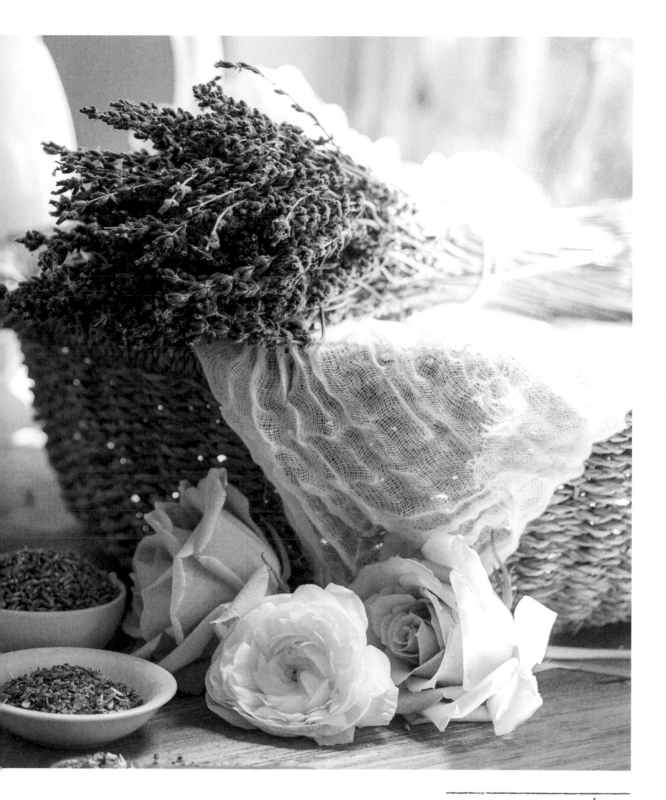

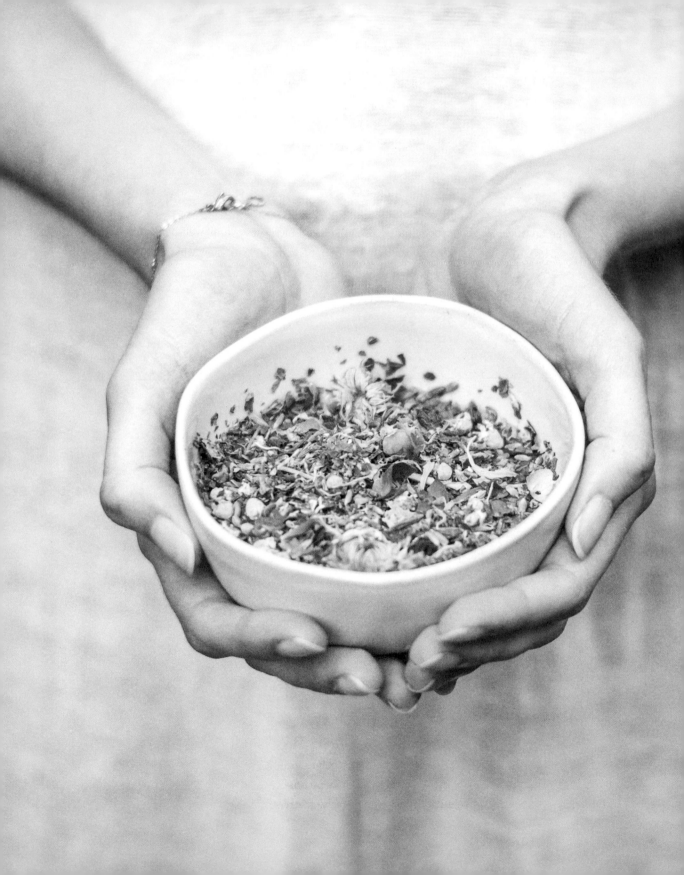

THE FIVE PILLARS
OF HEALTH

We've been talking a lot about food, and while we love to spend our days cooking and eating it's just not realistic—or healthy—to be only engaging with food. It is just one part of our life, and we should think of it as a means to ensuring that the rest of what we spend time on is fruitful, pleasurable, and sustainable. There are many ways to break down what constitutes our life in the macro and micro sense, but one model we find particularly helpful, and reflective of the holistic and integrated way we've found balance, is the Five Pillars of Health.

After reading through these categories, use the self-inquiry questions to examine where you fall on the spectrum of feeling balanced or imbalanced within the pillars. This is not meant to be a "quiz" where you get a score on how healthy you are, but rather a reflection of where you find yourself now, and a map for where you might want to go as you look to transform your habits and lifestyle. Then, take a look at the Root & Nourish Daily Rituals on page 220 for more specific ways to work with these concepts every day using herbs and self-care.

NUTRITION

Food is fuel for our bodies, and eating well is fundamental for our health. What you eat today affects the way you feel tomorrow and beyond. Eating a nutritious diet reduces the risk of diseases and increases overall well-being, but sometimes it is a struggle to know what that means or looks like. Lack of education about or access to nutritious foods can also impact our food choices. A good rule of thumb is to decrease consumption of processed and packaged foods, and foods high in added sugar, sodium, and saturated fats. Shop along the exterior perimeter of the grocery store, where most of the fresh, whole foods are available. Proper hydration is also essential for optimal wellness and is crucial to maintaining the function of every system in your body.

SELF-INQUIRY:

+ What foods do you eat most frequently during the week? Do you have cravings for certain foods? Are the cravings at certain times of the day or month?

+ Are you hungry for your meals?

+ Do certain foods cause you to feel discomfort after eating? If so, what are those, and how do they make you feel?

+ What is your energy level like after you eat? Do you feel satisfied and recharged after your meals?

+ Do you drink a sufficient amount of water daily, based on your needs and activity levels? Do you feel thirsty?

REST & SLEEP

Oftentimes we think rest and sleep are one and the same, but they have two distinct functions. Rest calms the mind, reduces stress, improves mood, and increases alertness. Sleep helps cell repair and regeneration, improves brain function and memory, and stabilizes the release of hormones, which regulate appetite and satiety, among other things. You can rest without sleeping, and sleep without resting—or, the goldilocks combination, rest while you sleep. When you don't get enough sleep, your metabolic and immune functions decrease, resulting in increased risk of illnesses.

It's recommended for adults to get seven to eight hours of sleep per night with two hours of rapid eye movement sleep (REM). The quality of sleep also matters. REM sleep is the most restorative of the sleep cycles, which is why we want more of it each night. We also need energy to sleep, since it is when important natural cleansing processes happen in the brain and throughout the whole body. What and when we eat therefore affect our sleep. Syncing our sleep to the rhythms of nature—known as our circadian rhythm—also ensures we get the best quality sleep our bodies are hungry for, which is why it's best to go to bed around 10 p.m. and wake up close to sunrise, around 6 a.m.

SELF-INQUIRY:

+ How many hours a night do you sleep? When do you go to bed and when do you wake up?

+ Do you have trouble falling asleep?

+ Do you wake up during the night? If so, for what reason, and for how long?

+ Do you wake up feeling rested?

+ Do you feel tired or fall asleep during the day?

MOVEMENT

Our bodies were not designed to sit in chairs all day—we live in a miraculous system of bones, soft tissues, muscles, nerves, blood, and more that work together in order to move. Daily movement is essential for health on a number of levels, and the lack of it is at the core of many chronic lifestyle diseases in our culture. Without movement, the natural flow of energy, nutrition, and the vital substances in our bodies can get disrupted, resulting in poor digestion and elimination, inflammation, altered mood and energy levels, imbalanced hormones (stress and reproductive), and acute and chronic pain.

Every body needs a different kind of movement, and we're not here to prescribe an exercise regimen to you. For most people, though, simple walking and some form of yoga, which incorporates physical and mental exercise, is safe and sustainable for long-term practice. Consider the quality and quantity of your movement on a daily and weekly basis, and where you might want to feed your body with motion.

SELF-INQUIRY:

+ What kind of movement do you engage in each day? Do you enjoy it?

+ What was your favorite type of movement when you were a child?

+ How do you feel after sitting for long periods, and how do you feel after exercise?

CONNECTION

We often think that optimal health falls mainly into the framework of the above-mentioned categories of nutrition, sleep, and movement—things that we more or less control individually. However, social connection is just as essential for wellness. Social connection improves physical, mental, and emotional well-being. It increases longevity, strengthens your immune system, and helps you recover faster from illness. There's also the connection we feel to natural beings—plants and animals—called "biophilia," and the lack of connection to the earth is yet another source of chronic illness. People who feel more connected to others, nature, and themselves report lower levels of anxiety and depression, and studies show that they have higher self-esteem, greater empathy for others, and are more trusting and cooperative.

SELF-INQUIRY:

+ Whom do you spend time with, and how do those beings make you feel?

+ How do you socially connect in a meaningful way?

+ When was the last time you had a social interaction that brought you joy?

+ How often do you spend time in nature?

+ Do you prioritize connection in your wellness routine? How?

SPIRITUALITY

Spirituality is a deeply personal and universal experience. Most of us can likely agree that we have felt a meaningful connection with something higher than ourselves at some point in our lives. However, the way we experience this feeling depends on many elements, such as our personal history, community, and the culture in which we live and were raised. While spirituality is broader than religion, the two are closely linked. Both may offer inner emotional peace in times of turmoil or hardship, give us a sense of our purpose, and invoke an awareness of reverence and wonder for the divine. Spirituality can provide better health and a longer life, coping skills in times of uncertainty and difficulty, and a sense of meaning and belonging.

SELF-INQUIRY:

+ Do you have a spiritual practice or routine?

+ When was a time you had a profound spiritual experience that brought you a sense of peace and clarity?

TOOLS FOR INTEGRATION

Our intention is to make the process of incorporating herbs into your life and diet as simple, intuitive, and accessible as possible. But any task, including ones that deal directly with nature, can be improved upon with the right tools. Below is a list of our staple kitchen equipment that make baking, blending, infusing, and storing these recipes more convenient—and more appealing to all the senses.

+ **BLENDER:** Regular or high-speed (like a Vitamix).

+ **DIGITAL KITCHEN SCALE:** Essential for weighing herbs and baking to ensure precision.

+ **ELECTRIC SPICE GRINDER:** For making spice blends and finer grinds of whole spices that the analog mortar-and-pestle method won't achieve. If you have a grinder for coffee beans, get yourself a separate one for spices/cooking so their distinctive scents and flavors don't cross.

+ **FINE-MESH SIEVES:** Having a variety of sizes will be useful for straining herbs and spices from liquids (teas, tonics, oils).

+ **FOOD PROCESSOR:** Can be used in place of a blender in most recipes and may be more appropriate for things like nut and seed butters where the ingredients are larger and/or harder to break down.

+ **FUNNELS:** For transferring liquids into bottles; have a variety of sizes for bottles with different-size mouths.

+ **GLASS STORAGE CONTAINERS WITH SCREW-TOP LIDS:** Clear glass mason jars with labels in a variety of sizes give your kitchen apothecary a uniform look and allow you to keep track of your ingredient stocks. Use them to hold dried herbs and spices, grains, legumes, nuts, and seeds. Keeping your leftovers, herb-infused oils and vinegars, and other prepared foods in glass also prevents by-products from plastics from leaching into your food, so it is helpful to Mother Earth as well.

+ **IMMERSION BLENDER:** A no-fuss tool for blending soups and other dishes in-pot, rather than transferring to a food processor or blender (and risking a messy explosion).

+ **MANUAL CITRUS JUICER:** You can certainly squeeze your lemons and limes by hand, but when they're part of your daily routine, having

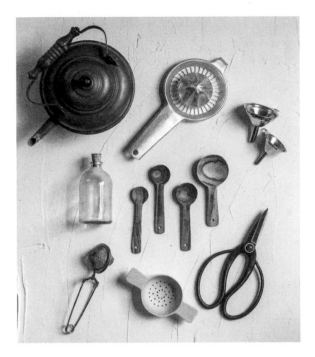

a tool to make juicing citrus easier can be a helpful (and pretty) addition to your kitchen.

+ **MORTAR & PESTLE:** Gently grinding herbs and spices with a mortar and pestle lets you engage all your senses in these ingredients' properties, so you really get to know your foods. It's also an attractive addition to your kitchen counter. For multiuse purposes, use a granite mortar with a wooden pestle, which has enough grit to work on tough spices (like cumin, coriander, and fennel seeds) but won't destroy delicate herbs like dried rose petals.

+ **NUT-MILK BAGS:** Designed to strain the pulp from nut milks (see our varieties on page 43), these mesh bags are multipurpose and reusable, though cheesecloth will work just as well if that's what you have.

+ **PARCHMENT PAPER & SILICONE BAKING MATS:** Earth-friendly liners keep your baking sheets from getting stained with burnt food

residue when roasting vegetables or making sweet treats. We encourage using reusable parchment (such as Super Parchment brand), which you can cut to whatever size you need and clean after each use. If you can't find reusable parchment, choose an unbleached compostable variety. Silicone baking mats (such as Silpat brand) are also great, but are less versatile when it comes to lining loaf pans and smaller baking sheets, and their slippery surface can cause baked goods like cookies (especially gluten-free ones) to spread.

+ **PRUNING SHEARS:** Save your regular scissors for paper and other things; shears made specifically for plants are useful for snipping off fresh leaves and flowers, especially from woodier stems like rosemary.

+ **STAND MIXER:** Makes whipping up baked goods fast and easy.

+ **TEA KETTLE OR SMALL POT WITH A LID:** A closed vessel is often useful for steeping teas and spices so their nutritive volatile oils don't escape.

+ **TEA INFUSER (ALSO CALLED A TEA BALL OR TEA EGG):** For steeping dry, loose-leaf tea in a mug or teacup of hot water or other liquid. Another option for loose tea is reusable tea bags. Look for bags made from organic cotton muslin; after use, simply empty the bag, rinse in the sink, then air-dry. All are sustainable alternatives to traditional disposable tea bags.

+ **THERMOS:** An Earth-friendly way of transporting teas and prepared meals, especially soups, and keeping them warm.

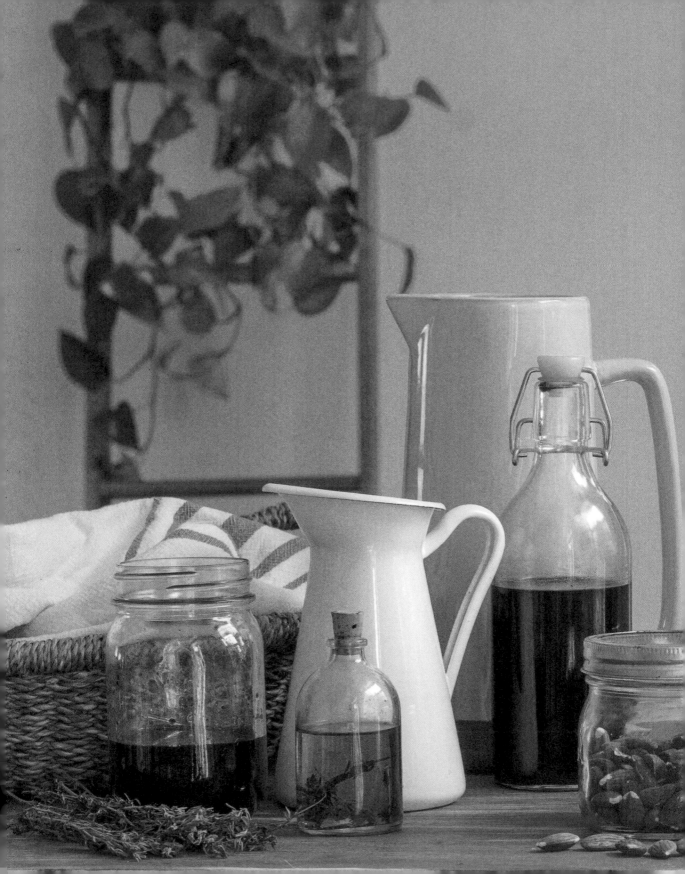

HERBAL PANTRY

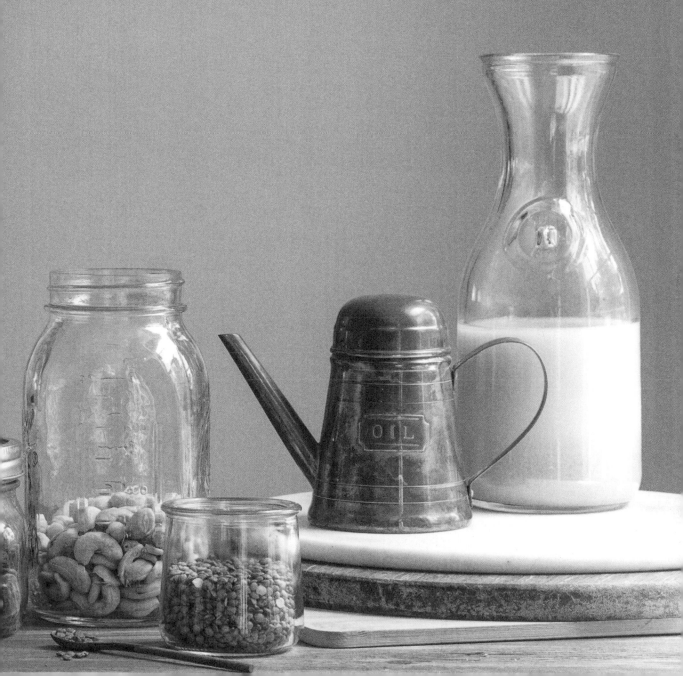

The key to long-term health is having a robust but simple foundation of staple foods and practices to keep you aligned with your true nature. With the herbs and tools listed in the Herbal Apothecary (page 23), you'll be well equipped to whip up any of the main dishes in this book. This section of Herbal Pantry items extends that tool kit to include the basic prepared ingredients we like to have on hand at all times. The more facility you gain with making these staple items, as opposed to relying on their processed and packaged versions, the closer your relationship with your food will be. Instead of needing to run out to the store for more almond milk or tahini or salad dressing, you'll be able to take care of those needs yourself, in the moment, and spend more time enjoying your meals and the people you share them with.

Like everything in this book, these basics are blank canvases on which you can create flavor and texture combinations that suit your personal tastes. If you're less experienced in the kitchen or are new to cooking with herbs, let these pantry items be your playground as you come to know which add-ins you like, as well as which methods and routines serve you best in keeping your home stocked with health.

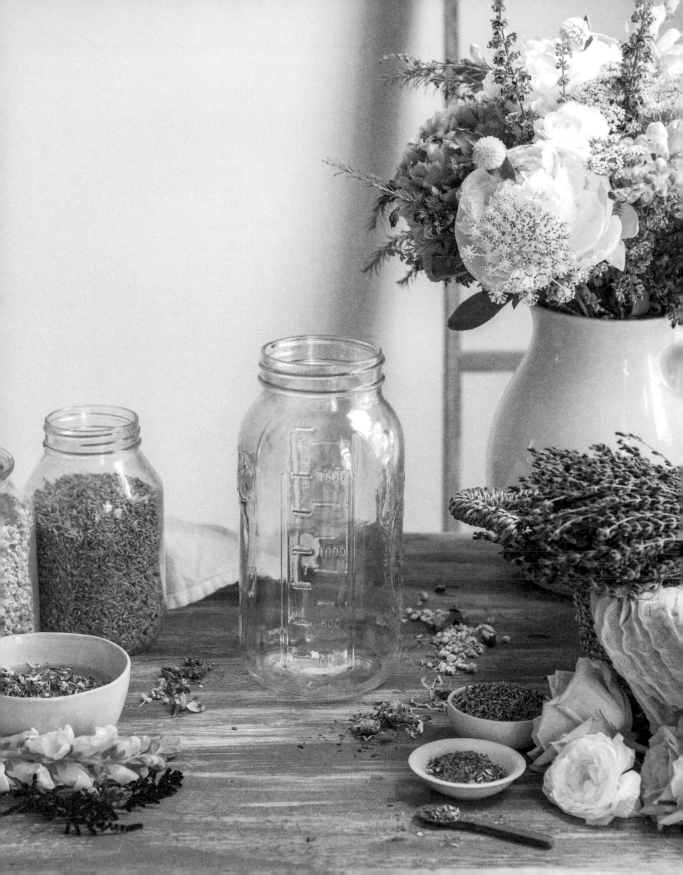

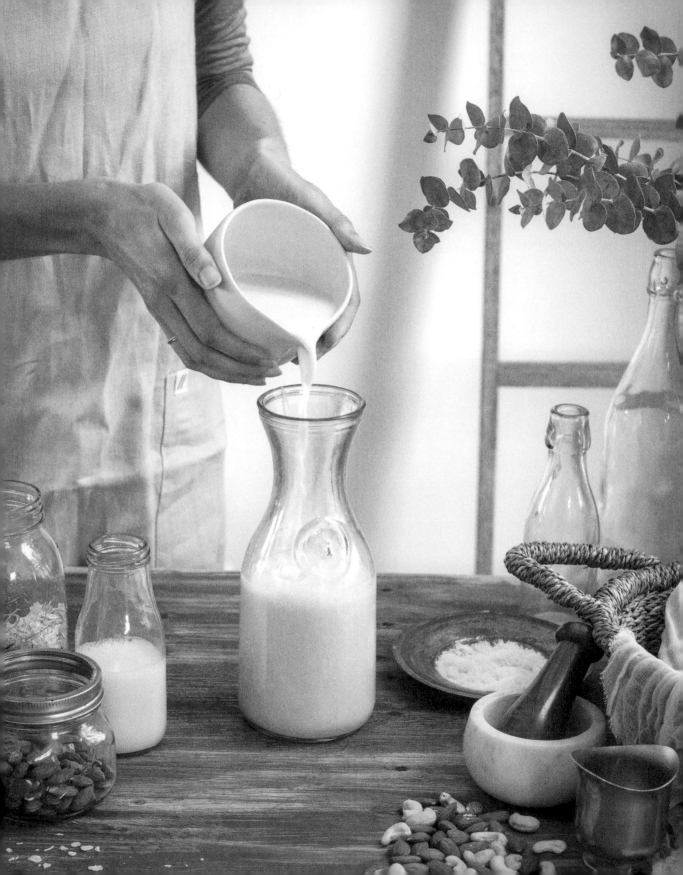

PLANT MYLK

PREP TIME: AT LEAST 8 HOURS, OR OVERNIGHT, SOAKING TIME   **COOK TIME:** 10 MINUTES   **MAKES** 4 CUPS

1 cup whole raw
   almonds or cashews,
   gluten-fee rolled
   oats, or unsweetened
   coconut flakes

1 Medjool date, pitted
   (optional)

Pinch of ground nutmeg
   (optional)

Pinch of pink Himalayan
   salt (optional)

Plant mylks may seem intimidating to make, but trust us it's the most fun you'll have in the kitchen, especially if it becomes part of your weekly food prep. Let your senses get into the process—there's nothing like milking your plants to really get to know them (especially oat mylk—try it then let us know how your hands feel). Once you get the hang of it, try a combination of nuts and grains—almond-oat and almond-cashew mylks are both delicious. Use these homemade mylks in the recipes throughout the book. We make recommendations for which plant is best for which dish, but feel free to interchange them or reach for a store-bought version in a pinch.

1. Soak the nuts or oats overnight, or at least 8 hours, in water to cover. (Coconut does not need soaking.) Drain, then put the almonds, cashews, oats, or coconut in a high-speed blender (see Notes). Add the date, nutmeg, salt, and 1 cup water (or, if making oat mylk, 1 cup of the reserved soaking liquid). Blitz until a light foam forms at the top, then add 3 cups more water, 1 cup at a time, and blitz until incorporated.

2. Strain the mylk through a nut-milk bag, cheesecloth, or a very fine-mesh sieve. Squeeze well to make sure all the liquid comes out. If using a sieve, set it over a bowl and strain the mylk by scraping and pushing on the solids with a spoon, letting the liquid collect in the bowl; then set a weight (like another heavy bowl) on top of the strainer and let rest for a few hours in the refrigerator.

3. Transfer the mylk to a widemouthed glass jar and cover tightly with a lid. Store in the refrigerator for up to 1 week. Since there are no added oils in this mylk, it will separate in the refrigerator—just give it a shake before using it.

NOTES: If you don't have a high-speed blender, you can blend the milk in batches using an immersion blender; work with ¼ cup soaked nuts or oats and 1 cup of water at a time.
   Save your solids! There are many fancy recipes out there for turning the pulp from mylked plants into cheeses, crackers, etc., but we love this simple way to make mylk a zero-waste staple. Simply spread the well-drained pulp on a baking sheet lined with reusable parchment and bake at 300°F for about 20 minutes, until golden and slightly crisped. Or spread the pulp in a thin layer in a large skillet, and cook over the lowest heat, tossing occasionally, until golden brown, crispy, and light, 15 to 20 minutes. It's great to sprinkle on a warm breakfast bowl, soup, or salad for a bit of crunch and texture.

VANILLA EXTRACT

PREP TIME: 10 MINUTES, PLUS AT LEAST 8 WEEKS SET TIME   **MAKES** 1 CUP

5 grade A or B vanilla beans

1 cup 80-proof alcohol, such as rum, vodka, bourbon, or brandy

Making your own vanilla extract is a more affordable and sustainable way to incorporate this robust flavor into your favorite recipes. By using top-quality vanilla beans, you cultivate a relationship with this ancient superfood, which is rich in antioxidants and nostalgia. Pure homemade vanilla extract lasts indefinitely and becomes more flavorful with time—the longer it extracts, the better the flavor becomes. You can really customize the flavor of your extract by the bean—depending on where they are grown, vanilla beans will have different notes, and most labels or descriptions will let you know what those flavors are. Spirits are commonly used for medicinal tinctures because of their optimal ability to extract the properties and flavors from herbal ingredients; for the alcohol base for this vanilla extract, rum, vodka, bourbon, and brandy all work well, and the spirit you choose will also affect the flavor of the extract. It's normal for the extract to have an alcohol smell initially. It will lessen over time and bakes out.

1. Split the vanilla beans lengthwise to release their oils and flavors, then chop them into pieces. Put the vanilla beans in a ½-pint mason jar with a lid.

2. Pour the alcohol over the vanilla beans, using a funnel to prevent any spilling. Secure the lid on the jar and shake well.

3. Store at room temperature in a dark place, such as in the pantry or a cupboard, for at least 8 weeks before using, to allow the vanilla to infuse the alcohol. Shake the jar every 2 to 3 weeks.

NUT & SEED BUTTERS

Making your own nut and seed butters is one of the most satisfying ways to replace store-bought pantry staples with homemade versions. While many tout the benefits of raw nuts and seeds, gently toasting them helps to enhance their robust flavor and brings out their natural oils, which we also want to unlock for the blending process. Sure, you could buy toasted nuts and seeds, but doing it yourself lets you know they're *freshly* toasted (because who really knows how long those bulk items have been hanging out on store shelves?). Plus, it makes your house smell delicious.

These three butters are used often throughout the book, but the general method can be applied to other nuts and seeds—cashews, peanuts, sunflower seeds, etc. Note that for roasting, larger nuts, like almonds or cashews, fare better in the oven than on the stovetop.

When you're blending, practice patience—the times we give aren't merely generalizations but the full amount of blending time required to get the butters super smooth and spreadable. And when you think you've blended enough, you could probably go a few more minutes. Dry, chunky nut butters are really not tasty, so: Blend. All. The. Way. (Pumpkin seeds may try your blending patience most of all, so be discerning of your mood when you go to make that butter.) Try mixing in spices and herbs in small quantities if you're feeling creative, but all on their own, these butters have powerful healing potential—seeds are, after all, the foundation for all life!

Nut butters (and whole nuts) can be taxing on sluggish digestive systems, but seed butters can be slightly lighter; tahini is the easiest to digest of all the varieties included here. If this condition applies to you, you might want to limit your consumption of these butters, or adjust the consistency by thinning them with a little bit of water when you're consuming them (but not while blending them).

STORAGE TIP: Store jars of nut and seed butters in the refrigerator upside down, to prevent oil separation, though we find that's less of a problem with homemade varieties than store-bought. You can store these butters in the refrigerator for up to 2 months (if they last that long!).

RECIPES FOLLOW

PUMPKIN SEED BUTTER

PREP TIME: 20 MINUTES   **COOK TIME:** 8 MINUTES   **MAKES** 1 CUP

2 cups raw hulled pumpkin seeds

Toast the pumpkin seeds in a large skillet over medium heat until golden brown and beginning to pop, about 8 minutes. Let cool to room temperature. Transfer the seeds to a food processor. Blitz for about 20 minutes (yes, it takes that long), stopping to scrape down the sides as you go, until the pumpkin seed butter is very smooth and a thin layer of liquid forms on the top.

TAHINI

PREP TIME: 30 MINUTES
COOK TIME: 25 MINUTES   **MAKES** 1¼ CUPS

3 cups hulled white sesame seeds

6 tablespoons to ½ cup extra-virgin olive oil or untoasted sesame oil (see Note)

Preheat the oven to 350°F. Line a baking sheet with reusable parchment. Arrange the seeds in an even layer on the baking sheet. Roast for 25 minutes, or until the seeds are just beginning to brown at the edges. Remove from the oven and let cool completely, for at least 20 minutes, then transfer the seeds to a food processor. Blitz for 2 to 3 minutes, until a rough crumble forms. Stream in the oil while you blitz for another 10 to 12 minutes, stopping to scrape down the sides as you go, until the tahini is very smooth and a thin layer of liquid forms on the top.

NOTE: Make sure you use hulled white sesame seeds for your tahini; brown seeds will make for a bitter, not-tasty spread. When it comes to the oil, you do need to add some for the best consistency (trust us, we tried it without). Choose plain sesame oil (which is golden in color), not the "toasted" variety (which is brown in color) that's often used in Asian cuisine. Olive oil makes for a lighter flavor, whereas untoasted sesame oil is quite nutty—see which you prefer, or use a combination!

ALMOND BUTTER

PREP TIME: 20 MINUTES   **COOK TIME:** 30 MINUTES
MAKES 2 CUPS

3 cups whole raw almonds

Preheat the oven to 300°F. Line a baking sheet with reusable parchment. Arrange the almonds in an even layer on the baking sheet. Roast for 30 minutes, then remove from the oven and let cool completely; the nuts will be slightly golden, not visibly crispy, but they will pop for a while as they cool. Transfer the almonds to a food processor and blitz for 10 to 15 minutes, stopping to scrape down the sides as you go, until the almond butter is very smooth and a thin layer of liquid forms on the top.

CASHEW CREAM

PREP TIME: 5 MINUTES, PLUS OVERNIGHT SOAKING **MAKES** 1 CUP

1 cup whole raw cashews

FOR SWEET CASHEW CREAM

2 teaspoons date syrup

1 teaspoon ground cinnamon

Pinch of flaky sea salt

FOR SAVORY CASHEW CREAM

2 tablespoons fresh lemon juice

1 tablespoon nutritional yeast

½ teaspoon sea salt

Scant ½ teaspoon garlic powder

¼ teaspoon ground turmeric

Simple yet versatile, this cream adds fluff and flavor to sweet and savory dishes alike—and is even delicious eaten straight out of the jar. We love to have a batch on hand all the time to dollop on soup, grains, sweet potatoes, and desserts. Enjoy it plain, experiment with the spice blends here, or create your own personalized cream flavor.

Put the cashews in a bowl and cover with 2 cups water. Soak in the refrigerator overnight. Drain the cashews and transfer to a deep bowl or wide-mouthed jar (if using an immersion blender) or a food processor. Add ½ cup fresh water and the sweet or savory add-ins (if using). Blitz until smooth. Store in a glass jar in the refrigerator for up to 5 days, or in the freezer for up to 1 month.

SOAKED DATES

PREP TIME: 10 MINUTES **MAKES** 2 CUPS

15 to 20 Medjool dates

Since dates are used so frequently in our kitchens, we like to have a stash of them ready for cooking and consumption at all times. Besides getting the dates nice and soft—which you'll want for the applications in this book—their soaking water (aka "date juice") is an excellent sweetener for drinks and sauces. (It's not quite thick enough to be a substitute for traditional date syrup, so we will indicate which you should use.) You can adjust the amount of dates you prepare based on how many you find yourself eating, but keep it to no more than two weeks' worth so they're fresh.

Split the dates in half, remove and discard their pits, then cut them in half again to make quarters. Put the quartered dates in a pint-sized glass jar or glass container with a lid. Pour in boiling water, submerging the dates completely, leaving a little bit of room at the top of the jar. Let cool to room temperature before covering with the lid. Store in the refrigerator for up to 2 weeks.

WHIPPED COCONUT CREAM WITH MARSHMALLOW ROOT

PREP TIME: 15 MINUTES, PLUS AT LEAST 3 HOURS OR OVERNIGHT SET TIME   **SERVES** 4 TO 6

1 tablespoon dried marshmallow root

1 cup full-fat coconut milk (see Note)

1 (13.5-ounce) can coconut whipping cream, chilled overnight (preferably Nature's Charm brand; see Note)

1 teaspoon pure maple syrup

¼ teaspoon pure vanilla extract, preferably homemade (page 44)

Marshmallow root is a demulcent herb, which means it is thick and slimy in texture and typically used to soothe mucous membranes. Combined with two forms of coconut—the milk it's infused in and the cream base for the whip—this topping is like a balm for your insides, cooling and moistening, bringing relief to hot and dry conditions. A spoonful is the perfect medicinal topping for nourishing treats or fruit, or all on its own.

1. Put the marshmallow root into a tea infuser. Place the tea infuser in a ½-pint mason jar with a lid. Pour the coconut milk over the infuser. Secure the lid on the jar and set in the refrigerator to infuse for at least 3 hours, or up to overnight.

2. Open the lid and remove the tea infuser. (It will be slimy due to the mucilaginous quality of the marshmallow root.) Using your thumb, press out any excess liquid from the marshmallow root; the extracted liquid will be a light tan color. Secure the lid on the jar once more and shake well to mix in the marshmallow root liquid.

3. Scoop the coconut cream into the bowl of a stand mixer and add 2 tablespoons of the marshmallow-coconut infusion. Store the remaining infusion in the refrigerator for up to 5 days (see Notes).

4. Whip the coconut cream on maximum speed for 2 to 3 minutes. Add the maple syrup and vanilla and whip for another 15 seconds, until combined.

5. Use immediately, or transfer it to an airtight glass container and store in the refrigerator to serve chilled. The whipped cream will naturally separate over time, so it is best used within 1 to 2 days. Rewhip before serving with a hand whisk if it deflates.

NOTES: For this recipe, you'll want to use pure liquid coconut milk, which is best found where you buy other plant-based milks (or make your own coconut mylk—see page 43). If you buy canned coconut milk, make sure to shake it well and pass it through a strainer to remove the thick, lumpy bits that usually float at the top.

If you can't find canned coconut whipping cream, you can make your own with full-fat coconut milk. Chill two cans in the refrigerator, which will consolidate the fats you use to make the cream. Don't shake the cans before you open them, and you'll be able to scoop out the cream from the top of the can. Use 1⅔ cups of the chilled cream for the recipe.

Leftover marshmallow root infusion can be used in tea or other drinks.

PLANT PARMESAN

PREP TIME: 5 MINUTES **MAKES** 2 CUPS

1 cup hemp seeds

½ cup raw walnuts

¼ cup nutritional yeast

2 tablespoons unsweetened coconut flakes

2 teaspoons umami spice blend (recipe follows)

Nondairy cheese substitutes are often riddled with chemical additives and fillers, which counteract the benefits of a plant-based diet. This homemade vegan cheese blend is perfect for sprinkling on your favorite savory dishes that call for a dash of umami, the flavor behind the sour-salty tang of Parmesan cheese, and a toothsome bite. Try it on soups or popcorn, or Heartwarming Vegan Chili (page 122), Mushroom Risotto (page 193), or Spinach Artichoke Cashew Dip (page 131).

Combine the hemp seeds, walnuts, nutritional yeast, coconut, and spice blend in a food processor and blitz until a coarse powder forms, 3 to 5 minutes. Transfer to a glass jar and store in the refrigerator for up to 1 month.

UMAMI SPICE BLEND

PREP TIME: 5 MINUTES **MAKES** ⅓ CUP

1 tablespoon reishi powder or mushroom blend powder

1 tablespoon dried thyme

2 teaspoons sea salt

2 teaspoons onion powder

2 teaspoons nutritional yeast

2 teaspoons dulse flakes

½ teaspoon garlic powder

½ teaspoon red pepper flakes

½ teaspoon freshly ground black pepper

Umami is known as the "fifth taste" in Western cuisine—a savory, full-bodied flavor naturally found in foods like mushrooms, tomatoes, and sea vegetables that delivers a satiating quality to your taste buds. Today, it's largely achieved in processed foods by the addition of MSG, but our spice blend lets you enjoy umami in a whole-food form. You can experiment with the ratio of herbs to meet your own personal taste, particularly if you're sensitive to spice and the red pepper flakes or black pepper is too much. Sprinkle some of this spice blend on hearty vegetables or legumes for extra support with digestion.

Combine all the ingredients in a small jar or spice shaker. Secure the lid and shake vigorously to combine well. Store in a cool, dry place for up to 6 months.

DRIED BEANS

PREP TIME: 8 HOURS OR OVERNIGHT   **COOK TIME:** 40 MINUTES   **MAKES** 2 CUPS

2 cups dried chickpeas

½ teaspoon baking soda

½ teaspoon hing

1 sheet kombu, broken into small pieces (see Note)

1 teaspoon extra-virgin olive oil

Beans can be tricky for many people's digestion: Their dry and astringent nature can make them hard to break down if the gut is stressed, overworked, or underworking. Cooking dried beans yourself is one way to mitigate the possible discomforts of these amazing plants; it also brings us closer to their natural form—always a good place to start (and stay) with foods to access their full nutritional profile. The combination of soaking and cooking for a *long* time offers important assistance to our guts, literally softening the hard beans so our stomachs work less to break them down. Adding baking soda and hing, a prominent Ayurvedic spice, contribute to this. Don't be scared of the hing—it's no coincidence that "fetid" is buried in its English name, asafoetida, since it has a rather pungent smell on its own, but when cooked it becomes mellow and umami. The kombu is another excellent source of umami flavor and trace minerals and vitamins that could be lacking in a vegan diet. While this recipe is for chickpeas, the method works for all medium or large dried beans, such as white beans, black beans, kidney beans, mung beans, and adzuki beans (smaller legumes like lentils don't need to be soaked prior to cooking, just give 'em a rinse to remove any debris and dust).

1. Place the chickpeas in a large bowl and add water to cover by about 2 inches. Soak in the refrigerator overnight. The beans will expand as they soak, so make sure you leave plenty of space in the bowl.

2. Drain and rinse the beans and transfer them to a large saucepan. Add 2 cups water, the baking soda, hing, and kombu. Bring to a boil. Once the water begins to foam on top, immediately reduce the heat to its lowest setting and drizzle in the olive oil to prevent boiling over. (If you think, "This is barely even cooking," you're at the right heat.)

3. Cover the pot with the lid slightly ajar. Cook the beans for 30 minutes, or until they are very soft (nearly falling apart) and their skins are blistering off.

4. Drain the beans in a fine-mesh sieve set over a wide bowl, reserving the cooking liquid in a jar. Remove the kombu, chop it into small pieces, and save it in an airtight container in the refrigerator for another use, up to 1 week.

5. Use the beans immediately or transfer them to a glass container, let cool to room temperature, and store in the refrigerator for up to 1 week. Store the reserved cooking liquid in a separate glass jar in the refrigerator or freezer; it's perfect as the base for a soup or a creamy dip, or as aquafaba (page 148).

NOTE: If you're preparing the beans for a recipe that needs a more neutral flavor (like the Cookie Dough Bites on page 197), leave out the kombu.

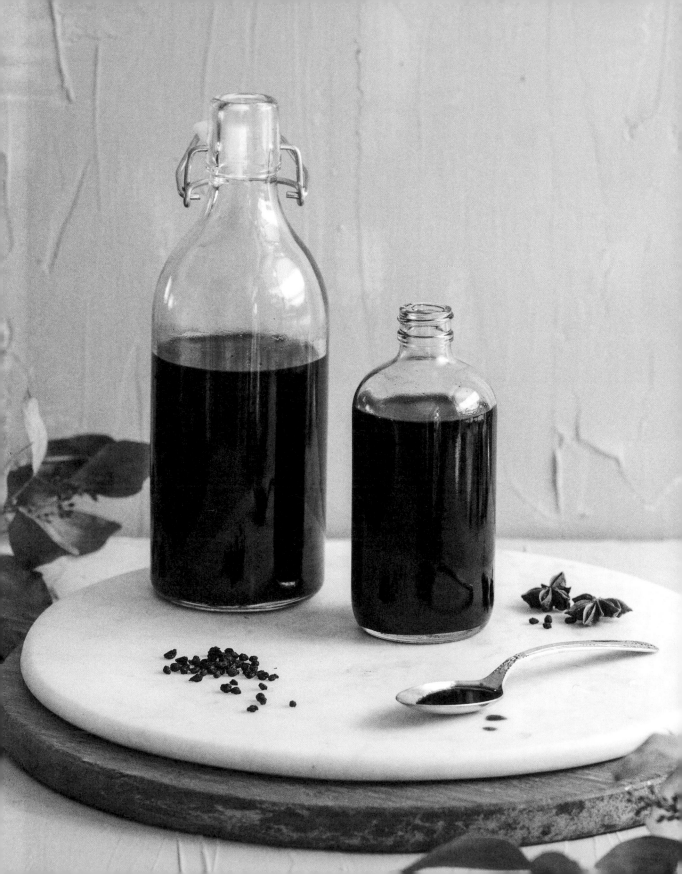

ELDERBERRY SYRUP

PREP TIME: 10 MINUTES   **COOK TIME:** 1 HOUR   **MAKES** 2 CUPS

¾ cup dried
   elderberries

5 whole cloves

1 cinnamon stick

1 star anise pod

1 cup raw honey

Elderberry syrup is a timeless herbal medicine traditionally used for colds and to support the immune system. It also makes a delightful syrup for drinks or topping for food. This syrup has a liquid consistency. If you want it to be more viscous in texture to use as a topping on pancakes or other desserts, mix ¼ cup elderberry syrup into 1 cup pure maple syrup or raw honey.

1. Combine the elderberries, cloves, cinnamon, and star anise in a large pot, and add 4 cups water. Bring to a boil over high heat, then reduce to medium and simmer for at least 1 hour, uncovered, until the liquid has reduced by half. Remove from the heat.

2. Strain the liquid through a fine-mesh sieve set into a large glass bowl, carefully pressing the solids with the back of a large spoon to extract all the liquid. Compost the solids and let the liquid cool, then stir in the honey.

3. Transfer the syrup to a glass bottle or jar. Store in the refrigerator for up to 3 months.

NOTES: It is *absolutely imperative* that the elderberries are cooked for a minimum of 1 hour, until the liquid has reduced by half. Consuming raw elderberries can pose serious health risks.

For adults, take 1 to 2 tablespoons daily to boost your immune system; take 3 to 4 tablespoons per day when sick. For kids, take ½ to 1 teaspoon per day for immune support, or 1½ to 4 teaspoons daily when sick.

HERBAL WATERS

Spice up your water with these flavorful herbal combinations to support a number of health needs. Simply add the herbs and spices to 4 cups boiling water, let steep, and sip throughout the day warm or at room temperature. You can strain out the herbs, if you wish, but it's no problem—even beneficial!—to ingest them as you drink.

WARMING DIGESTIVE WATER

1 (½-inch) piece fresh
    ginger, sliced

1 cinnamon stick

½ teaspoon ground turmeric

½ teaspoon raw honey
    (optional)

CLEANSING SPRING WATER

1 teaspoon ground ginger

1 cinnamon stick

1 teaspoon whole fenugreek
    seeds

Juice of ½ lime

DEEP HYDRATION WATER

4 cups coconut water

Juice of 1 lime

4 to 6 cucumber slices

COOLING SUMMER WATER

10 green cardamom pods

2 or 3 whole cloves

Pinch of whole fennel seeds

1 teaspoon fresh mint leaves (or ½ teaspoon dried)

1 teaspoon fresh food-grade rose petals (or ½ teaspoon dried rose)

ANYTIME DIGESTIVE WATER

1 teaspoon whole cumin seeds

1 teaspoon whole coriander seeds

1 teaspoon whole fennel seeds

HERBAL BALSAMIC VINEGAR

PREP TIME: 5 MINUTES, PLUS 1 TO 2 WEEKS INFUSING TIME   **MAKES** 2 CUPS

1 tablespoon dried
thyme

1 tablespoon dried
nettle

1 tablespoon dried
yarrow

2 cups balsamic vinegar

Herbal vinegar is a simple dressing for salads or fruit, or a dip for bread and herbal oil. The combination of thyme, nettles, and yarrow provides tonifying and healing medicinal properties to your basic balsamic vinegar.

1. Place the herbs in a clean 1-quart mason jar. Pour the vinegar over the herbs, submerging them completely. Secure the lid on the jar and let it sit in a cool, dry place for 1 to 2 weeks.

2. Strain the infused vinegar through a fine-mesh sieve into a glass jar. Optionally, you may use a funnel to transfer the herbal vinegar to a vinegar serving bottle. Store in a cool, dry place for 3 to 6 months.

<table>
<tr><td></td><td>

YARROW (ACHILLEA MILLEFOLIUM)
</td></tr>
<tr><td>

NOURISHING HERBS
</td><td>

Legend has it that yarrow was used to stop the bleeding of Greek warriors during the Trojan War (hence the yarrow genus is named after Achilles), but it also shows its prowess in supporting an easeful menstrual cycle for everyday female warriors. You may have seen its delicate white flowers in your neighborhood, as it's also a common weed, but this herb is no wallflower.
</td></tr>
</table>

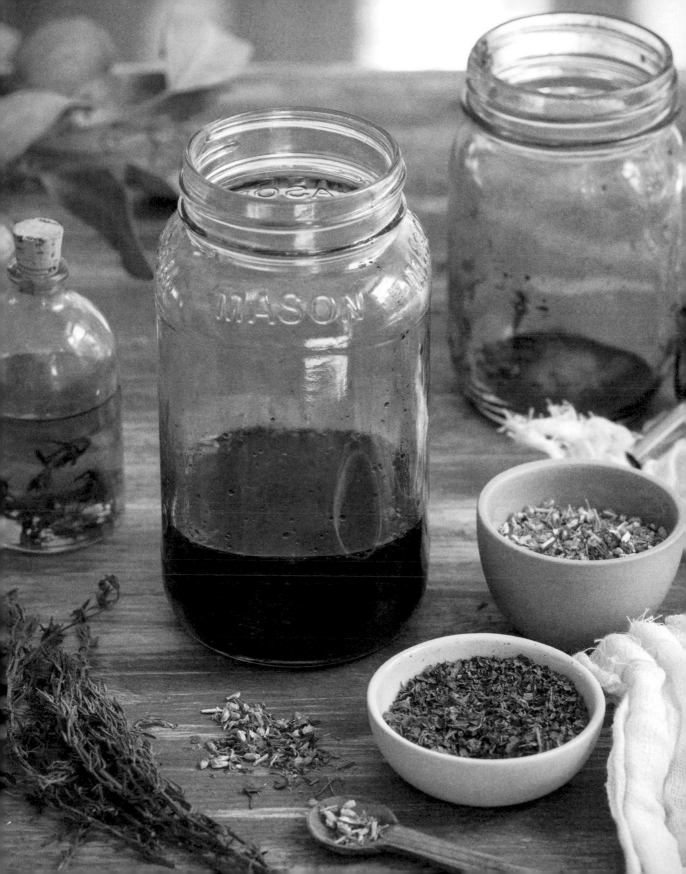

HERBAL COOKING OIL

PREP TIME: 5 MINUTES, PLUS 3 TO 6 WEEKS INFUSING TIME **MAKES** 4 CUPS

1 tablespoon dried yarrow

1 tablespoon dried chamomile flowers

1 tablespoon dried nettles

4 cups expeller-pressed avocado oil or extra-virgin olive oil

One of the easiest ways to harness the medicinal properties of herbs is using an herb-infused cooking oil. Expeller-pressed avocado oil and extra-virgin olive oil both cook well in high heat and can be used as a cold oil as dressing or dip. This combination of yarrow, chamomile, and nettle contains a wide range of healing actions and tonifying properties for overall wellness. Of course in a pinch, any of the recipes in this book can use regular avocado oil.

1. Place the herbs in a clean 1-quart mason jar. Pour all the oil into the jar, submerging the herbs completely. Secure the lid on the jar and let it sit on a windowsill for 3 to 6 weeks. Check regularly to make sure the oil is clean, and discard it if it becomes rancid (by smell) or moldy.

2. Set a nut-milk bag or a fine-mesh sieve lined with cheesecloth over a glass bowl. Strain the herb oil into the bowl, squeezing the bag or cheesecloth to extract as much oil as possible and letting it strain cleanly through the sieve. Using a funnel, transfer the oil to a clean mason jar, then secure the lid on the jar. Store in a cool, dry place for 3 to 6 months.

HERBAL VINEGAR BITTERS

PREP TIME: 5 MINUTES, PLUS 1 TO 2 WEEKS INFUSING TIME   **MAKES** 1 CUP

¼ cup dried dandelion root and leaf or any dried bitter herb of your choice

1 cup apple cider vinegar

Herbal bitters stimulate digestion and are best taken 10 to 15 minutes before mealtimes to get the digestive juices flowing. Combining bitter herbs with fermented apple cider vinegar provides beneficial gut bacteria and supports digestive wellness. Bitters can also be used in drinks, like our Passionflower Mocktail (page 149).

1. Place the dried dandelion in a clean ½-pint mason jar with a lid. Pour the vinegar over the herbs, submerging them completely. Secure the lid on the jar and let it sit in a cool, dry place for 1 to 2 weeks.

2. Strain the vinegar through a fine-mesh sieve into a clean glass jar. Using a funnel, transfer the herbal vinegar to a vinegar serving bottle. Herbal vinegar bitters can also be transferred to dropper bottles to easily take a small dose before a meal. Store in a cool, dry place for up to 3 months.

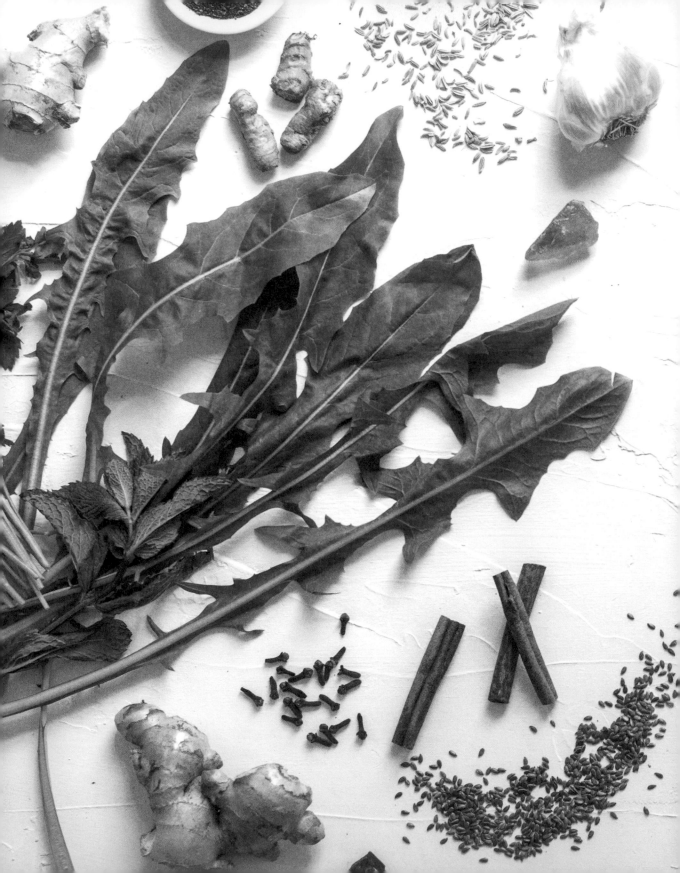

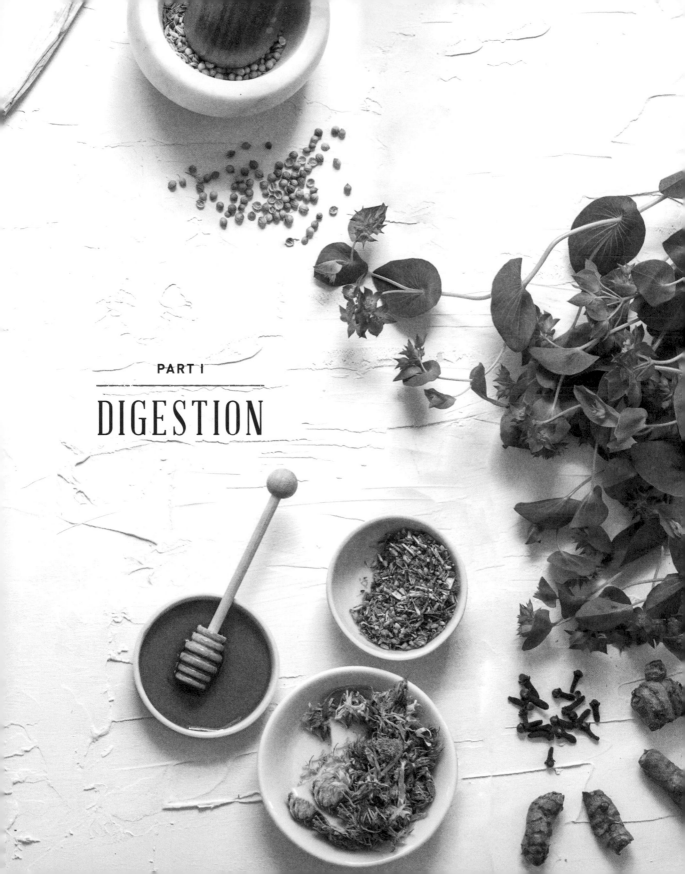

PART I

DIGESTION

> # When I began to eat
> # things happened.
>
> —MARY OLIVER, "THE MANGO"

You might think that in this section of the book, we'll be talking about digesting food—you know, the stuff you put in your mouth, chew, swallow, and eliminate in some way or another. That's true, but there's a lot more to digestion than just food. Holistic health traditions from all over the world identify digestion as the most important indicator of health, with impaired digestion being a primary factor in the cause of disease. If you've ever been to a holistic practitioner, you'll know that the first thing they ask about is your appetite, any taste in your mouth, and your bowel movements—which for Westerners can feel like a little TMI. But these conditions speak volumes about what you (body, mind, and spirit) have been taking in lately, and how all those parts of you are processing your food. The fact of the matter is, we're not just ingesting and digesting what we put in our mouths three (or more) times a day. We ingest and digest everything: people, information, the environment, external stimuli like noise and pollution, emotions, memories, and all the energy around us. The saying may go, "You are what you eat," but it's more accurate to say, "You are what you *digest*."

We could write entire books about the many faces of digestion (and many have already been written—head over to page 223 if you want to learn more), but in the context of this book, we'll stay within our scope and talk about how herbs can play a vital role in that vital process of digestion. Think about the last time your stomach was bothering you (maybe that's now), or you experienced constipation, diarrhea, acid reflux, or any of the myriad digestive issues out there. What were you able to concentrate on? What was your mood like? How did you feel about yourself? Most likely you were a little preoccupied with your discomfort, and suddenly everything else became secondary. That's why when people tell us they don't have the time or energy or interest to think about what they eat, we try to help them see it another way—it's when you *don't* think about what you eat that we suddenly have the time and mental space for nothing else.

On the flip side, when you're able to digest food properly, and absorb and assimilate all the nutrients of your food, everything else just starts to make sense. You feel better, so you're happier and your relationships improve. You bring more energy and creativity to your work. You start to see what really matters in your life and have the time to consider whether you're spending that time how and where you want to spend it. By investing just a few of your waking hours in preparing, cooking, and actually eating your food, you gain time back in spades, so you live more of your life in the present.

What to eat is no longer a secret (or particularly hard) to figure out: the whole-food, plant-based diet we share in this book has become mainstream, and is scientifically proven to increase longevity, balance mood and mental health, and prevent and sometimes reverse a host of chronic and acute illnesses. But if you don't pay attention to *how* you eat, too, even the healthiest meal on the planet won't do you any good. If you're surrounded by people who do not support your values, or if you have synced your jaw's chewing to your keyboard's clicking under the glow of fluorescent lights, you won't be digesting much. The environment in which we eat is as much a source of fuel (or not) as the food we're eating, so it's worth taking the time to clear the space around your meal physically and energetically.

Throughout this section, we include helpful tips for how to practice mindful eating, which involves simple things like not multitasking at meals, chewing your food thoroughly, and eating in silence (that doesn't mean alone, but it can). Note that "simple" does not mean easy, so if mindful eating is a struggle at first, just keep practicing. Doing so will maximize your food's digestibility and taste, so the more you do it, the more you'll enjoy your food . . . and the cycle continues from there. You'll learn to listen to your true cravings so it's easy to know what to eat, when to eat it, and how much to eat every day.

Food is also a way to shore up our intuition, particularly as women—by helping us connect to our bodies' natural cycles of hunger and satiety, recognize calm versus aggravated digestion,

and become mindful of responses to different ingredients. Eating healthy has never been the one-size-fits-all program many of us have been sold. Rather, the holistic models of herbalism and Ayurveda are based on personalization. Each of us needs to take responsibility for our health in all facets—what we call "integrative digestion." When we do this, we can derive even greater benefits from our food—a kind of nutrition for the spirit that will help us make better decisions that affect us and our communities, all throughout our lives.

The concept of integrative digestion has physiological aspects as well. Science shows that neurotransmitters located in the gut regulate everything from blood flow and nutrient absorption to hormone secretion and the stress response. By feeding our gut microbiome with healing herbs, we influence how we digest food and the stressors that impact our mind and reproduction, which we'll discuss in the other two sections of the book.

Where do herbs fit into this big, delicious world of digestion? Everywhere! Because herbs and spices contain the most potent concentrations of plant medicine, they can be incorporated into almost any main dish to support a specific condition or complaint, in addition to enhancing flavor with a literal pinch. The herbal actions relevant to digestion are below—refer back to page 26 for more about what they do.

+ Anti-inflammatory
+ Antimicrobial
+ Antioxidant
+ Antispasmodic
+ Astringent
+ Bitter
+ Carminative

+ Demulcent
+ Hepatic
+ Laxative
+ Tonic (digestive and liver)
+ Vulnerary

Within these actions, we'll be cooking with the specific herbs in the list on the following page. Take note of the overlaps and how the ingredients will support other areas of your well-being in addition to digestion.

You will find that the recipes in this section are deliberately on the conservative side when it comes to spices. This is because, for the most part, we are addressing the needs of sensitive or compromised digestive systems—and using gentler, fewer, and more targeted spices is the first step to getting back into balance. Spices are very healing, but if you're unable to digest them, their medicinal aspects will go to waste, and may actually have a toxic effect on the body. If you have a healthy GI, though, and/or a palate acclimated to these flavors, please feel free to increase the spices and personalize accordingly. Remember, the body will often ask for what it needs, so if it's asking for a full teaspoon of cinnamon instead of a quarter teaspoon, go for it!

Outside of herbs and spices, certain foods are also essential to any gut-friendly pantry, whether you're maintaining your digestion or working to regulate it. Fermented and cultured foods are potent sources of prebiotics and probiotics, which support the growth of good bacteria in the gut and throughout the whole body. Science is discovering the increasing importance of our microbiome—turns out, we are 90 percent bacteria!—and how integral it is to maintaining every system of the body (nervous, cardiovascular, respiratory, digestive, etc.), as well as its role in immunity, reproductive function, physical fitness, balanced mood and mental health, and even supple, radiant skin. Our favorite plant-based ferments (and preferred brands/varieties), which appear throughout this section, include:

+ **Coconut yogurt:** Anita's or GT's CocoYo
+ **Kimchi:** Mother-in-Law's
+ **Miso:** Miso Master, South River
+ **Olives**
+ **Pickles**
+ **Sauerkraut:** buy it from your local farmers' market if available
+ **Tempeh:** Lightlife
+ **Vinegar (white, balsamic, apple cider):** Bragg (for apple cider vinegar)

Remember, as you build your herbal digestive tool kit, start slowly. Experiment with the recipes that address your current digestive problems or that just look good to you. Your unique makeup will have a unique response to everything you eat, so if one ingredient is throwing you off, change it! We won't mind, promise. If you take the time to get to know your gut and really listen to it, you might find that the menu of things that nourish you—foods as well as experiences—takes on a whole new flavor.

ASHWAGANDHA (*WITHANIA SOMNIFERA*)	anti-inflammatory, astringent
BASIL (*OCIMUM BASILICUM*)	antispasmodic, carminative
BLACK PEPPER (*PIPER NIGRUM*)	antioxidant, carminative (alpha)
CALENDULA (*CALENDULA OFFICINALIS*)	anti-inflammatory, antimicrobial, antispasmodic, vulnerary
CARDAMOM (*ELETTARIA CARDAMOMUM*)	carminative
CAYENNE (*CAPSICUM FRUTESCENS/ANNUUM*)	antimicrobial, antioxidant, antispasmodic, carminative
CHAMOMILE (*MATRICARIA CHAMOMILLA*)	anti-inflammatory, antimicrobial, antispasmodic, bitter, carminative, vulnerary
CHIA SEED (*SALVIA HISPANICA*)	demulcent
CHICORY (*CICHORIUM INTYBUS*)	aperient, bitter, digestive tonic, hepatic, laxative
CILANTRO (*CORIANDRUM SATIVUM*)	anti-inflammatory, carminative
CINNAMON (*CINNAMOMUM ZEYLANICUM*)	antimicrobial, antioxidant, astringent, carminative
CLOVE (*SYZYGIUM AROMATICUM*)	antimicrobial, antioxidant, carminative
CUMIN (*CUMINUM CYMINUM*)	anti-inflammatory, antispasmodic, carminative
DANDELION ROOT AND GREENS (*TARAXACUM OFFICINALE*)	bitter, digestive tonic, hepatic
ELDERBERRY (*SAMBUCUS NIGRA* SUBSP. *CANADENSIS*)	anti-inflammatory, antioxidant, antispasmodic, aperient, carminative
FENNEL (*FOENICULUM VULGARE*)	anti-inflammatory, carminative
FLAXSEED (*LINUM USITATISSIMUM*)	anti-inflammatory, aperient, demulcent
GARLIC (*ALLIUM SATIVUM*)	antimicrobial, antispasmodic, carminative
GINGER (*ZINGIBER OFFICINALE*)	carminative, laxative
HING (*FERULA ASSA-FOETIDA*)	antispasmodic, carminative
LICORICE ROOT (*GLYCYRRHIZA GLABRA*)	anti-inflammatory, antispasmodic, demulcent, hepatic, laxative, liver tonic
MARSHMALLOW ROOT (*ALTHAEA OFFICINALIS*)	demulcent
PARSLEY (*PETROSELINUM CRISPUM*)	carminative
PEPPERMINT (*MENTHA PIPERITA*)	anti-inflammatory, antispasmodic, carminative
PSYLLIUM (*PLANTAGO PSYLLIUM*)	aperient, demulcent, laxative
REISHI (*GANODERMA LUCIDUM*)	anti-inflammatory, antioxidant, hepatic
TURMERIC (*CURCUMA LONGA*)	anti-inflammatory, antioxidant, astringent, digestive and liver tonic
YARROW (*ACHILLEA MILLEFOLIUM*)	anti-inflammatory, antispasmodic, astringent, digestive and liver tonic, vulnerary

AVOCADO SAUERKRAUT TOAST

PREP TIME: 5 MINUTES   **SERVES** 1

1 slice gluten-free bread

2 tablespoons White Bean Beet Hummus (page 184) or other hummus

½ avocado, sliced

2 to 3 tablespoons sauerkraut

Pink Himalayan salt, to serve

First there was PB&J, peas and carrots, bread and butter: now we have avocados and toast. If you're an avocado toast aficionado, this recipe will elevate your experience of the now-staple. With the addition of tangy sauerkraut, the creamy avocado-and-hummus base gets a probiotic boost that naturally supports a healthy whole-body microbiome even as it delivers light yet filling nutrients and minerals.

Toast the bread and let it cool for about 1 minute (otherwise the toppings will melt). Layer with the hummus, avocado slices, and sauerkraut. Season with salt as desired, and enjoy immediately.

WEEKDAY CHIA SEED PUDDINGS

PREP TIME: 5 MINUTES, PLUS 5 HOURS OR OVERNIGHT TO SET   **SERVES** 1

The best things come in small packages, and the incredible chia seed is no exception. These mighty mucilaginous superfoods are just what any inflamed gut needs for a healing coating of calm, comfort, and regularity. You can enjoy these five chia puddings throughout the day, and every day of the week, but they make an especially nice breakfast during warmer seasons, and are perfect for nutrition on the go. The complementary ingredients in these varieties—cacao, coconut, and all the spices—also add helpful pre- and probiotics for microbiome support.

CALMING VANILLA & OATS

¾ cup almond mylk, preferably homemade (page 43)

2 tablespoons pure maple syrup

¼ teaspoon pure vanilla extract, preferably homemade (page 44)

2 tablespoons chia seeds

2 tablespoons gluten-free rolled oats, for topping

PROBIOTIC ELDERBERRY

¾ cup almond mylk, preferably homemade (page 43)

2 tablespoons pure maple syrup

1 tablespoon Elderberry Syrup (page 53)

½ teaspoon psyllium husk powder

¼ teaspoon ground cinnamon

¼ cup chia seeds

½ cup coconut yogurt, for topping

SAVORY GREEN GODDESS

¾ cup coconut milk

1 tablespoon green curry paste

¼ teaspoon ashwagandha root powder

¼ teaspoon sea salt

¼ cup chia seeds

2 tablespoons chopped cashews, for topping

DOUBLE CHOCOLATE CACAO

1 cup almond mylk, preferably homemade (page 43)

2 tablespoons pure maple syrup

1 tablespoon raw cacao powder

½ teaspoon reishi powder

¼ teaspoon ground cinnamon

¼ cup chia seeds

CHAI THIS

¼ cup almond mylk, preferably homemade (page 43)

2 tablespoons pure maple syrup

¼ teaspoon ground cinnamon

¼ teaspoon ground ginger

¼ teaspoon ground allspice

⅛ teaspoon ground cardamom

¼ teaspoon pure vanilla extract, preferably homemade (page 44)

¼ cup chia seeds

METHOD FOLLOWS

1. In a glass jar or container, whisk together all the ingredients except the chia seeds and toppings until smooth.

2. Add the chia seeds and stir.

3. Cover and refrigerate for at least 5 hours or overnight, until set and a gelatinous consistency.

4. When you're ready to eat, stir the pudding to mix together the flavors. Then add the suggested topping, if desired, and serve cold.

NOTE: If you prefer your pudding more gelatinous, you can reduce the liquid to ½ cup; alternatively, if you prefer a looser consistency, increase the liquid to 1 cup. Remember to stir your pudding after its first night in the refrigerator before eating it to reincorporate any liquid that separated out and to give the pudding an even texture.

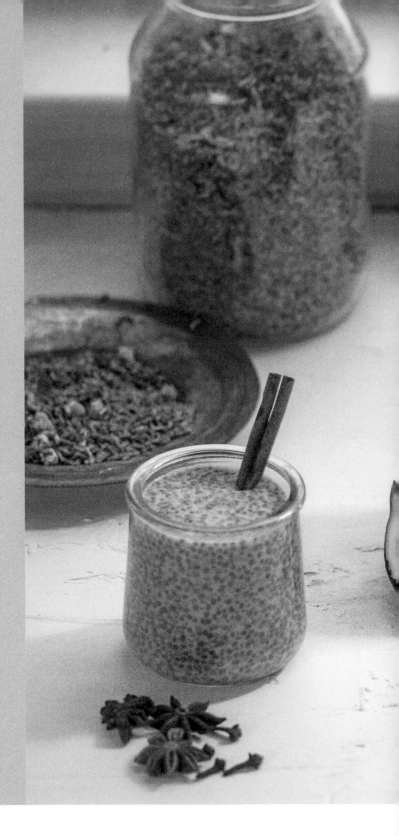

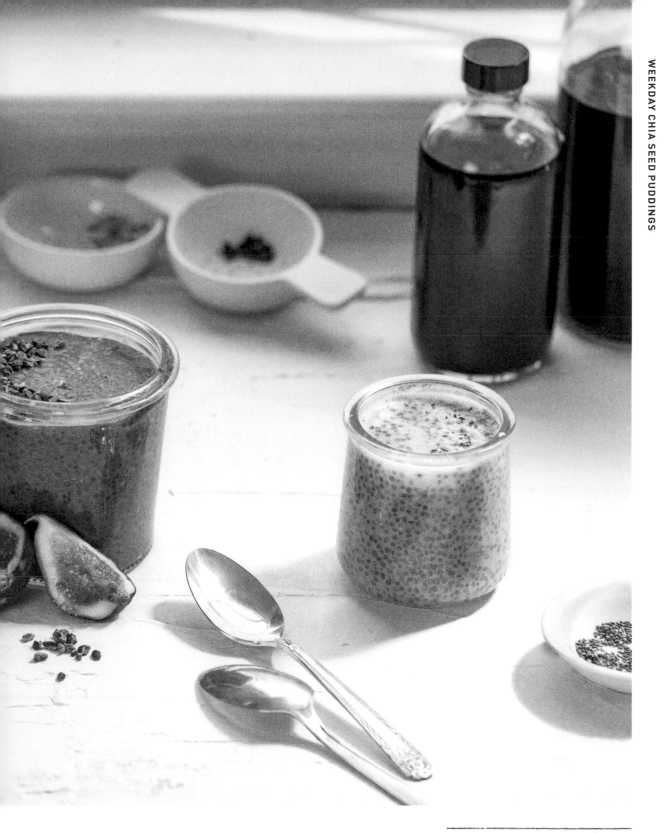

ESSENTIAL BANANA BREAD MUFFINS

PREP TIME: 15 MINUTES   **COOK TIME:** 25 MINUTES   **MAKES** 12 MUFFINS

2 tablespoons flax meal

1¼ cups gluten-free measure-for-measure flour blend (King Arthur Brand preferred)

¾ cup almond flour

½ cup gluten-free rolled oats

1 tablespoon baking powder

1 teaspoon baking soda

1 teaspoon ground cinnamon

½ teaspoon sea salt

3 ripe bananas (the uglier and browner the skin, the sweeter the muffin)

¼ cup pure maple syrup

¼ cup extra-virgin olive oil

3 tablespoons apple cider vinegar

1 teaspoon pure vanilla extract, preferably homemade (page 44)

1 cup coconut sugar

½ cup chopped raw walnuts (optional)

Bananas are nature's fast food: they come in their own container, can be eaten neatly while ambulating by foot or otherwise (though we don't recommend that . . . !), and are as perfect on their own as they are when paired with creamy nut butters or decadent chocolate. In a muffin form, they may be even more delectable, and keep you going for longer with their fiber-filled flax, oats, and walnuts. Coconut yogurt adds a satisfying, lightly sweet flavor to these can't-have-just-one breakfast bites. They may even draw you and your family to the table for a sit-down breakfast, whether for five minutes or an hour, during which the real digestive magic will take place.

1. Preheat the oven to 375°F. Line a 12-cavity muffin pan with compostable unbleached paper liners or lightly grease with coconut oil.

2. Stir together the flax meal and 6 tablespoons hot water in a bowl and let stand for about 5 minutes, or until thickened (see Note).

3. Meanwhile, combine the flours, oats, baking powder, baking soda, cinnamon, and sea salt in a medium bowl.

4. Add the bananas to the mixer bowl with the flax. Stir well by hand or with a hand-mixer until the bananas are well mashed and broken down into a more liquid form (some small chunks of banana may still be visible). Add the maple syrup, olive oil, vinegar, vanilla, and ¾ cup of the coconut sugar. Mix well until thoroughly combined.

5. Slowly add the dry ingredients into the bowl and stir until the batter just barely comes together; do not overmix, which will result in dense muffins. Stop and scrape down the sides of the bowl as needed.

6. Pour the batter into the prepared muffin tin, filling each cavity to the top. Sprinkle the tops evenly with ¼ cup coconut sugar and walnuts, if desired. Bake for 25 minutes, until the tops are golden brown. Remove from the oven and let rest in the tin for 5 minutes. Turn the muffins out of the tin and serve. Store in an airtight container in the refrigerator for up to 3 days.

NOTE: Flax meal is often sold pre-ground in stores, but since these seeds have volatile oils just like any others, making your own will ensure its freshness. Use your spice grinder to pulverize whole, golden or brown flaxseeds into a coarse meal, and store the meal and whole seeds in an opaque container (to prevent the light from oxidizing the seeds) for up to 1 month in the refrigerator or freezer. Preparing these seeds monthly is a great way to support your Lunar Rituals as well (page 176).

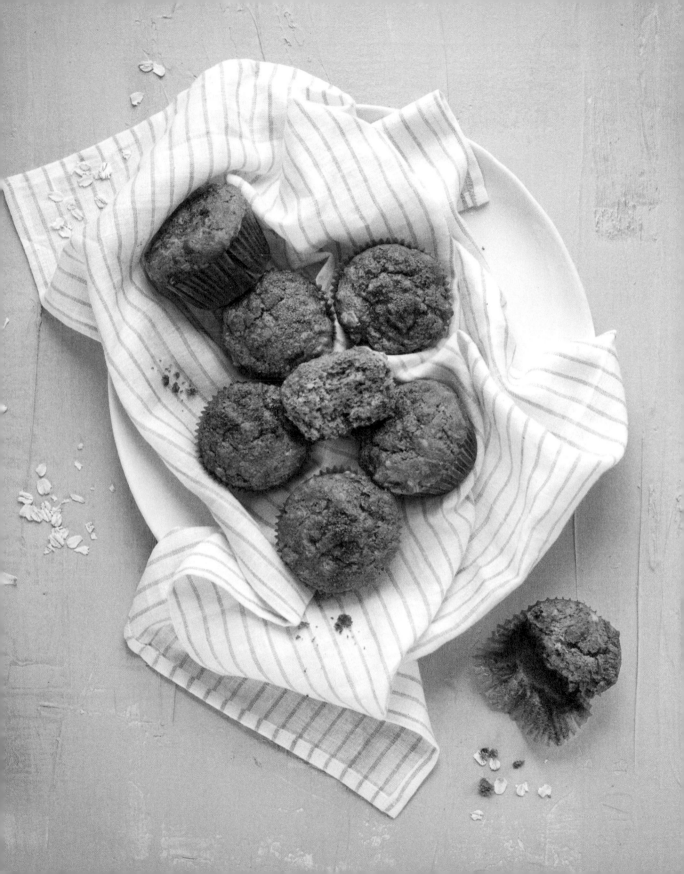

THE RULE OF THREES FOR ROOTED DIGESTION

When we're trying to be conscious of our health, it's easy to put a lot of time and effort into what we eat (you are holding a cookbook, aren't you?). But if we don't think about how we eat, even the healthiest meal can be indigestible and undigested. It may seem (or actually be) impossible to sit down at a calm, elegantly set table for every meal, but easeful digestion is as simple as counting to three. Follow the Rule of Threes each time you eat to create the conditions your body needs to integrate all the healing love and nutrition you put into your meal.

3 Breaths: Before your first bite and after your last, pause and take three full, long breaths. Start by bringing your attention to the surface that you're sitting on. As you breathe in, let the air expand your whole torso, into the sides of your ribs and all the way down into your lower belly and pelvis. Allowing the mind and the body to reset and come into the present moment through slow, mindful breathing activates the parasympathetic nervous system, which is responsible for the "rest and digest" functions of the body. If we try to eat while the sympathetic nervous system ("fight or flight") is turned on, our bodies' energies are too focused on survival mechanisms (i.e., craving sugar for explosive, short-term energy), and our metabolism slows.

3 Meals: Skipping meals or frequent snacking can seem appealing or necessary if you're dealing with digestive woes. However, having fewer, nutrient-dense meals evenly spaced throughout the day optimizes hormonal function and digestion. Larger meals also allow for more mindful eating; putting together a well-balanced plate (or bowl) requires more attention and takes longer to eat than snacks that you can pop in your mouth while multitasking. If you're used to snacking, it may take a while for your system (body and mind) to adjust, so have compassion if you make the meal transition gradually.

3½ to 4½ Hours Apart: We all know not to swim after eating, and the same principle applies to . . . more eating! The body needs time to break down, process, and eliminate what you've given it, so allowing 3½ to 4½ hours between meals provides ample time for digestion and a hormonal reset. If you're constantly snacking, your body is always being asked to produce insulin, which throws off the metabolic process and doesn't let the body return to homeostasis during the day (or even at night, depending on when you're snacking). This time frame fits squarely into the 3 Meals rule: If you have breakfast at 8, lunch at 12:30, and dinner at 5, you have 12-plus hours between your first meal and your last meal, which also keeps your circadian clock running on schedule. This may be challenging to incorporate into your social or work routines, so again be patient and do your best. If your relationships depend on late-night gatherings, see if you can make them less about eating and more about quality time, like games or just talking.

CHAMOMILE MOONG DAL PORRIDGE

PREP TIME: 5 MINUTES **COOK TIME:** 35 TO 40 MINUTES **SERVES** 2

- ½ cup dried moong dal (split mung beans)
- ½ teaspoon ground ginger
- ½ teaspoon ground cardamom
- ¼ teaspoon ground turmeric
- 1 teaspoon loose chamomile tea or 1 chamomile tea bag
- ½ teaspoon coconut oil
- 4 dried figs (¼ cup), quartered
- 1 cup chopped apples
- 2 tablespoons unsweetened coconut flakes or chips
- 2 teaspoons raw honey

Oats have their place in every herbal cook's day, but even the most ardent oatmeal fan needs a break from time to time. This warm, creamy, non-grain dish is a heartier, more toothsome alternative to the classic warm breakfast cereal. On its own, moong dal (the Hindi name for split mung beans) might come off as savory, and you can follow that impulse by adjusting the spices or add-ins. The sweeter variety in this recipe is more useful for irregular and inflamed digestion, especially for constipation and bloating. Cooking the fruit in the dal will help improve its digestibility, but the simplicity of the dal on its own, sans fruit, can also be delightful when the stomach is overwhelmed. By cooking the dal in what is basically chamomile tea (or a chamomile stock, if you fancy that), you'll also get a breakfast that both stimulates the appetite and encourages digestion, as this potent herb has bitter and carminative herbal actions. Wake up right with this symphony of gut support!

1. Rinse the dal two or three times, or until the water runs clear, then transfer it to a medium saucepan. Add the ginger, cardamom, turmeric, chamomile tea (placed in a tea infuser, if you are using loose tea), and 1½ cups water. Bring to a boil, then reduce the heat to low. Add the coconut oil (this prevents the dal from boiling over) and cover loosely.

2. After 10 minutes, add the figs and apples. Cook for another 15 minutes without stirring. Once the apples are mushy and the dal has absorbed all the water, remove from the heat and let cool for 5 to 10 minutes, uncovered. Remove the tea infuser or tea bag and stir in the coconut.

3. Ladle the porridge into two bowls. Drizzle each with 1 teaspoon of the honey and serve.

BERRY PROBIOTIC AÇAI BOWL

PREP TIME: 5 MINUTES **SERVES** 1

1 (3.5-ounce) packet frozen açai smoothie purée (preferably Sambazon)

¼ cup coconut water

1 frozen peeled banana

¼ cup almond butter, preferably homemade (page 47)

½ cup quartered strawberries

½ cup raspberries

¼ cup raw hulled sunflower seeds

1 tablespoon chia seeds

1 tablespoon hemp seeds

1 teaspoon ashwagandha root powder

2 tablespoons coconut yogurt (optional)

If the saying is true and you are what you eat, then eating this colorful, flavorful, and healthful bowl will bring out every ounce of your natural inner beauty—and help your gut work beautifully, so you are what you digest, too. Chia seeds reign supreme when it comes to mucilaginous foods, which support healthy elimination while soothing any inflammation along the gastrointestinal tract. Combined with fruits rich in prebiotics (banana) and probiotics (berries), this hydrating and refreshing bowl is ideal for restoring an appreciation for the many healing aspects of food.

1. Place the açai, coconut water, and frozen banana in a blender and blitz until smooth. Pour the purée into a bowl.

2. Spoon the almond butter into a small glass dish and microwave on high for 15 to 20 seconds, or set the bowl in a larger dish of boiling water to warm for a few minutes, until the almond butter is runny.

3. Top the açai purée with the strawberries and raspberries. Drizzle the almond butter on top and sprinkle with the sunflower seeds, chia seeds, hemp seeds, and the ashwagandha powder and coconut yogurt, if using. Serve immediately.

NOTE: Confused about what kind of bacteria you need for an optimal whole-body microbiome? As their name suggests, prebiotics support the gut microbiome *before* we get to the actual intestines. They're found in foods (plant fibers, technically) that support the growth of good bacteria, including just about all produce containing complex carbohydrates, such as fiber (leafy greens, chicory root, dandelion greens, garlic, onion, and asparagus are among the best sources). On the other hand, probiotics enter the game *after* digestion is underway. They are live organisms that will support an existing colony of bacteria and can be found in fermented foods including plant-based sources like tempeh, tofu, sauerkraut, kimchi, and coconut yogurt. Aim to have a variety of both in your diet to make a happy gut—and a happy life.

SMOOTHIE SEASON

Cold, creamy fruit purées like smoothies can be difficult to digest, especially first thing in the morning, and are not generally recommended by Ayurveda. The exceptions are when excessive heat is present—such as during the summer, when the sun is high in the sky at midafternoon and digestion is strongest, or if you have an inflammatory condition. In these cases, you may wish to enjoy your smoothie bowl as a warm-weather treat, rather than in fall and winter, or as lunch instead of breakfast.

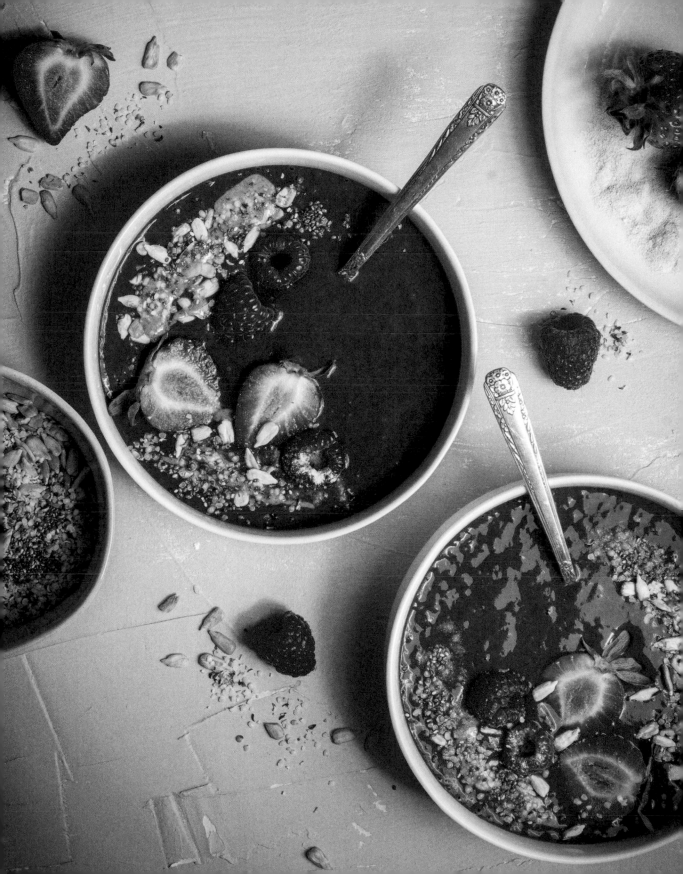

SLOW & SIMPLE CONGEE

PREP TIME: 30 MINUTES SOAKING TIME **COOK TIME:** 1 HOUR **SERVES** 4

1 cup uncooked white basmati rice, soaked for 30 minutes

1 sheet kombu

½ to ¾ teaspoon grated fresh ginger

¼ teaspoon ground turmeric

When it comes to medicinal foods, congee reigns supreme in the less-is-more approach. Varieties of this porridge exist in many Asian cultures, which attests to the universality of its healing properties. Hulled basmati rice, cooked down to a soupy, sticky consistency, acts like a soothing balm for the digestive system and delivers a balanced proportion of carbohydrates and protein without making your gut do a lot of work. Kombu (a variety of seaweed) and ginger complement this nutritive action with healing minerals and anti-inflammatory and antibloating properties—plus, they add a bit of flavor to the otherwise bland rice, whetting your appetite as well.

Congee is a perfect way to balance a day or period of inconsistent or indulgent eating, before or after travel, or after eating many different kinds of foods or flavors at once (like you might during the holidays), which can confuse and overwhelm the gut. It's great just on its own, or combined with a handful of mix-ins, whether savory (steamed greens, roasted veggies, baked tofu) or sweet (stewed apples, dates, coconut) for a heartier meal.

Drain the rice, then rinse it two or three times, until the water runs clear. Transfer it to a large pot and add the kombu, ginger, turmeric, and 8 cups water. Bring to a boil over medium heat, then reduce the heat to maintain a simmer, cover, and cook for about 1 hour, until the rice is very thick. Do not stir. Remove the kombu and discard it, or chop it into pieces and stir it back into the congee to serve.

NOTE: Congee is best eaten fresh, but if you need to keep leftovers add a bit of water as you reheat it. It's an excellent dish to use for a monodiet (page 82), and this recipe will satisfy you for an entire day's worth of meals; simply leave the pot on the stove and scoop out your congee whenever you're ready to eat throughout the day. It is safe to leave out of the refrigerator for 24 hours.

COCONUT FENNEL CASHEW CURRY

PREP TIME: 15 MINUTES, PLUS 30 MINUTES SOAKING TIME   **COOK TIME:** 40 MINUTES   **SERVES** 4 TO 6

TOASTED CASHEW TOPPING

½ cup raw cashews, coarsely chopped

1 tablespoon whole fennel seeds

1 (1-inch) piece fresh ginger, peeled and finely chopped

½ cup unsweetened coconut flakes

1 cup uncooked white basmati rice, soaked for 30 minutes

3 teaspoons sea salt, plus more for serving

2 teaspoons whole fennel seeds

1 teaspoon whole coriander seeds

1 teaspoon whole cumin seeds

1 tablespoon untoasted sesame oil or extra-virgin olive oil

1 teaspoon ground turmeric

1 (½-inch) piece fresh ginger, grated

1 ([16]-ounce) block firm tofu, pressed and cubed (see Note)

Traditional curries are known for their vibrant blends of spices, which can spell disaster for an irritated belly. This recipe turns down the heat a few notches by featuring ingredients that are more soothing but just as flavorful. With its mild incorporation of all the tastes (Ayurveda identifies six: sweet, sour, salty, pungent, bitter, and astringent) and a variety of textures (creamy, crunchy, chewy), this curry is perfect to serve when picky eaters (adults and children) are around the table, too. Set up a toppings station where people can personalize their bowl, and you'll have a fully harmonious meal.

1. Make the cashew topping: Toast the cashews, fennel seeds, and ginger in a dry large skillet over medium heat for 2 minutes. Reduce the heat to low, add the coconut, and toast for another 3 to 5 minutes, moving the seeds and coconut around in the pan a few times until the coconut is browning and the mixture is fragrant. Transfer to a plate and set aside.

2. Drain the rice, then rinse it two or three times, until the water runs clear. Combine the rice, 2 teaspoons of the salt, and 1¾ cups water in a large pot. Bring to a boil over medium heat, then reduce the heat to low. Cover and simmer for 20 minutes, until the water has been absorbed and the rice is soft. Remove from the heat, place a paper towel under the pot lid, cover again, and let rest for 10 minutes. (The paper towel will absorb any extra moisture, making the rice nice and fluffy.)

3. Lightly grind the fennel, coriander, and cumin seeds with a mortar and pestle, or gently crush them between your two hands. In the same skillet you used for the topping (it will already be warm), combine the sesame oil with the ground spices and toast on low heat for 5 minutes, or until just beginning to brown and become fragrant. Stir gently, then add the turmeric and ginger and cook for another 2 minutes.

4. Add the tofu and the remaining 1 teaspoon salt to the pan, and stir gently to coat the tofu in the spice mix without crumbling it. Cook for about 8 minutes, without disturbing the tofu, until the tofu begins to brown (not stirring will help it cook more evenly and prevent it from crumbling).

INGREDIENTS & RECIPE CONTINUE

¼ cup full-fat coconut milk

½ cup pure pumpkin purée

¼ cup Plain or Savory Cashew Cream (page 48; more for serving, optional)

1 small fennel bulb, chopped (about 1 cup)

½ bunch spinach, coarsely chopped or torn (2 to 3 packed cups)

½ cup chopped fresh cilantro, leaves and stems, for garnish

Lime wedges, for serving

5. Combine the coconut milk, pumpkin, and cashew cream in a small bowl, and stir to combine. Add the mixture to the pan with the tofu. Stir gently to combine, then cook for about 3 minutes, until warmed.

6. Add the chopped fennel bulb. Stir to combine with the tofu and cream mixture, then cover and cook for 10 more minutes. Add the spinach, cover, and cook for 3 to 5 minutes, until the greens are wilted.

7. To serve, spoon the rice into bowls and top with generous portions of the curry. Season with additional salt, if desired, then garnish with the cashew topping and cilantro and serve with the lime wedges alongside for squeezing.

NOTE: Pressing tofu ensures this plant-based protein maintains a dense and toothsome texture. Simply wrap the tofu in a paper towel or tea towel, set inside a strainer over a bowl, and weigh down with another bowl, can, or glass you have on hand. Let sit for at least 10 minutes, up to 1 hour. Remove the paper towel and give the tofu one more squeeze over the sink before preparing to cook. You can also freeze the whole block of tofu right in the package and follow the same steps to press for a spongier, "meatier," texture.

BELLY YOGA

Bite, chew, swallow, poop, repeat. Digestion is a rather miraculous mechanical process that, thankfully, happens all on its own all day long—most of the time. If your system is getting clogged somewhere along the way, these gentle yoga postures can help get things moving again by assisting the downward passage of food through your GI tract, called peristalsis.

SQUATS: Start your day off right on both feet with some gentle squats. Stand with your feet hip-distance apart and your weight over your heels. Bring your hands to your hips. As you breathe in, bend at your knees and ankles, sitting backward as if into an imaginary chair. Breathe out to return to standing. Go as deep into the squat as is comfortable for your joints; take a wider stance with your feet if you have any tension in your lower back. Do 10 to 20 reps, at a pace that feels invigorating but not strenuous. Notice if there are any changes in your bowel movements during the day.

SIT: Take a simple cross-legged seat (a posture known as *sukhasana*) while you eat. It may take a while to ditch your chair habit but sitting with the legs close to the body will help direct energy to the digestive organs in your gut, rather than sending it outward to your extremities. Sitting in any position while eating is *always* preferable to standing or walking. If sitting cross-legged is uncomfortable, try propping your pelvis up on a pillow or folded blanket, or using support under your knees.

LSD & WALK: Ayurveda recommends a two-step, post-digestion routine that helps to support peristalsis. After your meal, take a few breaths and lie with your left side down (LSD) for 10 to 15 minutes; this will encourage food to move into the stomach. You can also "lean" to the left if you're unable to lay down fully. Then take a gentle 10- to 15-minute walk (not a power walk or jog)—preferably outdoors (indoors is fine, too). Try a simple walking meditation where you say the word "place" silently to yourself each time you take a step. This will encourage a sense of grounding and slower gait that your body needs to digest well.

PROBIOTIC QUINOA CABBAGE STIR-FRY

PREP TIME: 15 MINUTES   **COOK TIME:** 40 MINUTES   **SERVES** 4 TO 6

¾ cup uncooked quinoa, rinsed

1 sheet kombu, torn into thin strips

1 teaspoon plus 1 tablespoon untoasted sesame oil

1 tablespoon white hulled sesame seeds

2 tablespoons unsweetened coconut flakes

1 tablespoon tamari

1 tablespoon grated fresh ginger

2 garlic cloves, grated

1 (16-ounce) block firm tofu, pressed and cubed (see Note, page 78)

1 (10-ounce) container baby bella or white mushrooms, sliced (see Note)

1 small bunch radishes, leaves chopped (1½ cups) and radishes sliced (about 1 cup)

½ head napa cabbage, cored and chopped (3 cups)

Zest and juice of 1 lime

1½ teaspoons white miso paste

2 tablespoons apple cider vinegar

1 cup kimchi, chopped

½ teaspoon ground turmeric

Overflowing with probiotic foods, this bowl is the perfect way to transition through and out of any gut disturbance, whether it's from poor dietary patterns, antibiotics, or stress. From the fermented foods to the kombu to the mushrooms, which get a little boost from the limes' vitamin C, these bold flavors are cooked long and slow to make them mellow and easy to digest.

1. Combine the quinoa, kombu, and 1½ cups water in a medium pot and bring to a boil over high heat. Reduce the heat to low to maintain a simmer, add 1 teaspoon of the sesame oil (to prevent boiling over), and cover. Cook until the quinoa is tender, about 10 minutes. Remove from the heat, place a paper towel under the lid, cover again, and let rest for 5 minutes. (The paper towel will absorb any extra moisture, making the quinoa nice and fluffy.) Remove the kombu strips, and either discard them or chop them up to mix into the quinoa when serving. Fluff the quinoa with a fork.

2. While the quinoa is cooking, toast the sesame seeds and coconut in a large skillet over low heat until golden and fragrant, 2 to 3 minutes. Transfer to a small bowl and set aside for garnish.

3. In the same skillet, combine the remaining 1 tablespoon sesame oil, the tamari, ginger, and garlic. Stir just to combine, then cook over low heat for 2 to 3 minutes, or until the garlic is browning and fragrant.

4. Add the tofu and toss to coat in the sauce. Cook over medium-high heat, turning the tofu occasionally, for 10 minutes, or until it begins to brown. Add the mushrooms and radish slices. Cover and cook for 20 minutes.

5. Meanwhile, in a separate sauté pan, combine the cabbage and radish greens with ¼ cup of water and cook over medium heat, uncovered, for 10 minutes, or until the greens have begun to wilt slightly but are still bright. Remove from the heat, add the lime zest and a squeeze of lime juice, and stir.

6. Whisk together the miso and vinegar in a small bowl with a fork. Add the mixture to the pot with the quinoa, then add the kimchi and turmeric and stir well to combine.

7. To serve, spoon the quinoa into bowls and top with the vegetables and tofu. Garnish each bowl with additional lime juice and lime wedges and the toasted sesame seeds and coconut.

RESTORATIVE KITCHARI

PREP TIME: 10 MINUTES, PLUS 30 MINUTES SOAKING TIME   **COOK TIME:** 40 MINUTES   **SERVES** 4

½ **cup uncooked white basmati rice, soaked for 30 minutes**

½ **cup dried moong dal (split mung beans), rinsed**

1 **teaspoon ground turmeric**

¾ **teaspoon mineral salt (see Note)**

½ **teaspoon hing**

1 **cinnamon stick, or 1 teaspoon ground cinnamon**

6 **whole green cardamom pods, lightly crushed, or ½ teaspoon ground cardamom**

2 **to 6 cups chopped mixed vegetables (carrots, broccoli, spinach, cauliflower, and/or sweet potato, chopped into small, even pieces; optional)**

TARKA
1½ **teaspoons cumin seeds**

1½ **teaspoons coriander seeds**

½ **teaspoon fennel seeds**

1 **tablespoon untoasted sesame oil or extra-virgin olive oil**

1 **tablespoon grated fresh ginger**

Kitchari is a traditional Ayurvedic medicine for any and all digestive troubles, including many of the other imbalances that arise from disturbed digestion. The main ingredients, basmati rice and moong dal (split mung beans), are extremely easy to digest, since the tough outer shell of the rice (which is left intact in brown rice) is removed and the tiny dal kernels are already split—essentially, much of the work your body would need to do to digest the dish is already done for you, so the nutritious carbohydrates and proteins can get into your system without asking too much of your GI tract.

Generous helpings of spices and herbs transform this kitchari from basic to craveable. Turmeric, one of the best anti-inflammatory herbs, gets mixed into the grains and given a nice, slow simmer. Hing, a traditional Indian spice ground from a dried plant resin, removes the potential gassiness of the beans and lentils. (When you smell hing, known as asafoetida in English, you'll understand how it got the nickname "devil's dung"! Don't worry, though: the odor becomes a mellow and earthy taste when cooked, but you may wish to store your jar of hing inside another glass container in your cupboard.) Ayurveda's triple threat—coriander, cumin, and fennel (see Note)—form the base of the tarka, a tempering of spices that lets their essential oils bloom on their own before they're mixed into a dish. Adjust the spices according to your taste and digestion—use less if you're feeling very irritated or if you're new to Indian cooking. The same goes for the vegetables: start with no vegetables, or fewer of them, if you are feeling very imbalanced, and add more as you begin to heal.

---

1. Drain the rice, then rinse it two or three times, until the water runs clear. Combine the rice, dal, turmeric, salt, hing, cinnamon, and cardamom in a large pot and add 4 cups water. Bring to a boil over medium heat, then reduce the heat to low. Cover and simmer, without stirring, for 20 minutes. Check to see if the kitchari is drying out; if it is, add 1 cup more water.

2. Meanwhile, make the tarka: Lightly grind the cumin, coriander, and fennel seeds with a mortar and pestle, or gently crush between your two hands. Warm the sesame oil in a skillet over medium heat for about 1 minute. Add the ground spices and the ginger, and stir to coat. Reduce the heat to low, and cook until the spices are fragrant, about 5 minutes. Be sure to watch the tarka, as the spices can burn easily. Remove from the heat and set aside.

3. If using the vegetables, add them to the pot with the kitchari. Stir gently to combine, and cover for another 10 to 15 minutes, until the dal and vegetables are very soft, like a porridge.

INGREDIENTS & RECIPE CONTINUE

TO SERVE

½ cup chopped fresh cilantro (see Note)

1 lime or lemon, cut into wedges

Mineral salt (see Note)

Freshly ground black pepper

4. When the kitchari is done, add the tarka to the pot and stir just to combine.

5. Serve with the cilantro and a squeeze of lemon or lime juice, and season with salt and pepper, as desired.

NOTES: Cilantro stems are the most medicinal part of this cooling herb, so don't let them go to waste!

Mineral salt is a form of pink salt with trace minerals, such as iron, magnesium, and calcium (and sodium, too), that are essential to the body's functions. It is generally easy to digest and does not cause as much water retention as other salts. Salts with these naturally occurring minerals are more healthful and restorative to the body, as opposed to common table salt. Be conscious of where your salt is sourced, since the abundance of pollution in our oceans has resulted in salts laced with microplastics. If you're confused about which salt to use in any of our recipes, know that mineral salt, sea salt, and Pink Himalayan salt will all work interchangeably—so there's no need to season your food with anxiety!

Having a jar of premixed cumin, coriander, and fennel seeds (whole, not ground or toasted) on hand is a great way to be always prepared for kitchari—as well as for Ayurvedic CCF Tea (page 98). If you're in a digestive pinch, simply take a few of the seeds in your mouth, chew, swallow, and let the gut-pacifying begin.

KITCHARI AS MONODIET

Kitchari is often recommended as a one- to five-day monodiet to rest the body when imbalanced, or during seasonal transitions, when we are more susceptible to illness. This recipe can be enjoyed anytime, including as part of a short at-home reset. When following a monodiet, you eat the same dish for every meal—in this case, a single pot of kitchari will probably be enough to get you through one day. Try to limit your other activities (work, socializing, exercise) and enjoy more periods of rest and relaxation. If you are experiencing severe or chronic digestive imbalances, please consult a doctor or holistic practitioner before beginning a monodiet.

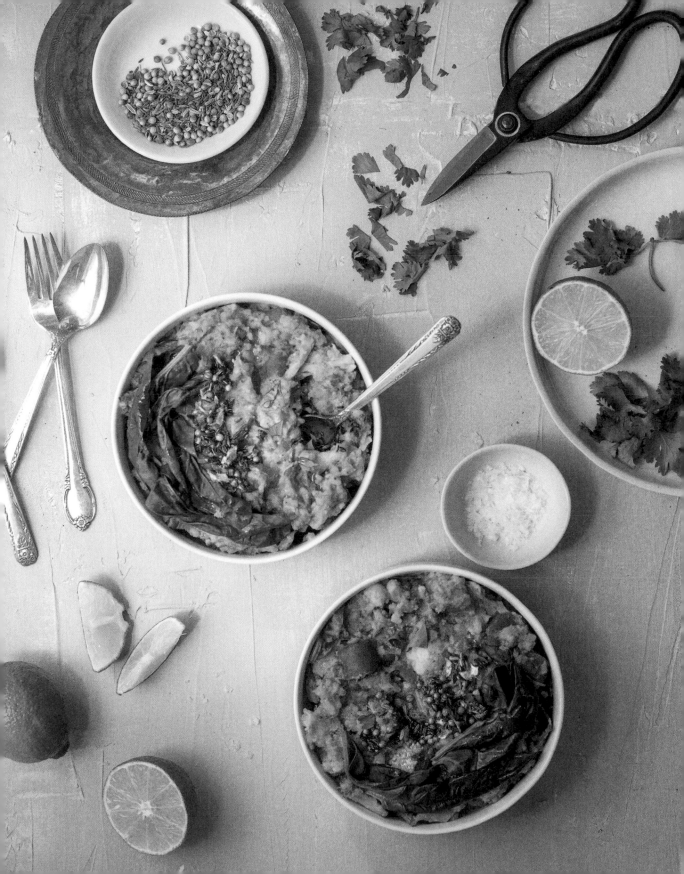

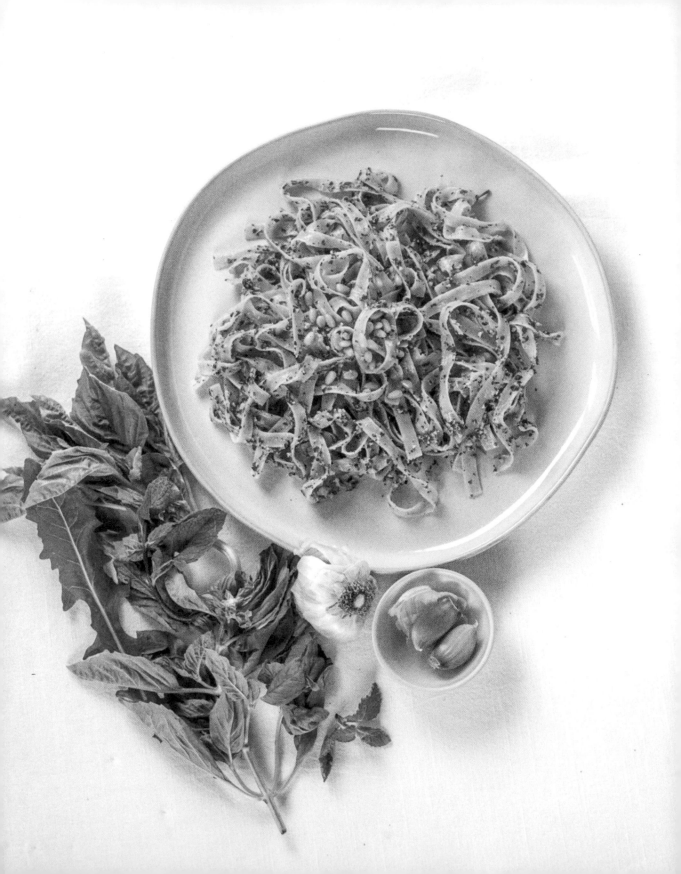

WILD DANDELION & MINT PESTO

PREP TIME: 10 MINUTES   **SERVES** 2 TO 4

½ cup pine nuts

1 garlic clove, peeled

1 tablespoon Plant
  Parmesan (page 50)

1 teaspoon nutritional
  yeast

1 cup fresh basil

½ cup fresh dandelion
  greens

½ cup fresh mint leaves

1 tablespoon lemon zest

1 tablespoon fresh
  lemon juice

½ cup extra-virgin
  olive oil

1 teaspoon sea salt

When you think of pesto, you probably envision the classic basil dish. However, pesto can be much more imaginative when you invite other nourishing greens and herbs into the mix. Dandelion is a popular bitter to stimulate digestion, making it an excellent addition to the pesto. Paired with the cooling and carminative properties of mint, this pesto is a burst of slightly bitter and vibrant flavors. Since both these greens grow abundantly in the wild during the spring and summer seasons and are easily foraged, this meal also connects us more fully to the earth, allowing us to feel its life-giving qualities deeply. Combined with other healing spices, nuts, and oils, this pesto is delicious on anything that needs a sauce or dip—gluten-free pasta, steamed lentils, or cooked vegetables.

Combine the pine nuts, garlic, parmesan, nutritional yeast, basil, dandelion greens, mint, lemon zest, lemon juice, olive oil, and salt in a food processor. Process until smooth. Serve immediately or transfer to a glass jar or airtight container and store in the refrigerator for up to 4 days.

NOTE: If you prefer a less bitter pesto, add another tablespoon of fresh lemon juice and more salt. These flavors will naturally counteract the bitterness. If the pesto is too thick for your liking, pour in more olive oil 1 tablespoon at a time, until it reaches your desired consistency.

CHUNKY FENNEL, BEET & CHICKPEA SALSA

PREP TIME: 30 MINUTES   **SERVES** 3 TO 4

1½ cups cooked or canned chickpeas (see page 51)

1 garlic clove, grated

1 tablespoon apple cider vinegar

1 teaspoon horseradish mustard

1½ cups diced fennel bulb and stalks (about ½ bulb), fronds reserved

1½ cups diced beets

¼ cup finely chopped fresh parsley

Sea salt and freshly ground black pepper

Normally, raw foods are not recommended for anyone suffering from digestive ailments, since the high fiber in most plants can tax an already overworked system. In this refreshing, crunchy, and colorful salsa, the stomach gets a break, thanks to some manual breaking down of the ingredients—i.e., chopping. Take your time to finely dice the vegetables—if you struggle with slowing down, then this recipe is also a powerful exercise in mindfulness.

The ingredients are paired for a reason, too. Fennel plus the soaked and well-cooked beans relieve and prevent bloating; the beets feed your microbiome; and the parsley finishes each bite with a cooling, light flavor to balance the sweetness and umami of the other ingredients. Enjoy this salsa chilled, at room temp, or even warm—the texture and flavors are so versatile that it pairs just as easily with a hearty chip at a backyard picnic as it does spooned over lightly steamed greens for a salad, used as a delightful pita filling, or straight out of the bowl!

1. Place 1 cup of the chickpeas in a food processor and pulse five or six times to coarsely chop them.

2. In a small bowl, whisk together the garlic, vinegar, and mustard.

3. Combine the fennel and beets in a large bowl. Add the chopped chickpeas and the remaining ½ cup whole chickpeas. Add the garlic dressing, parsley, and ¼ cup of the reserved fennel fronds; stir everything gently to avoid mashing the chickpeas.

4. To serve, season with salt and pepper and top with additional fennel fronds.

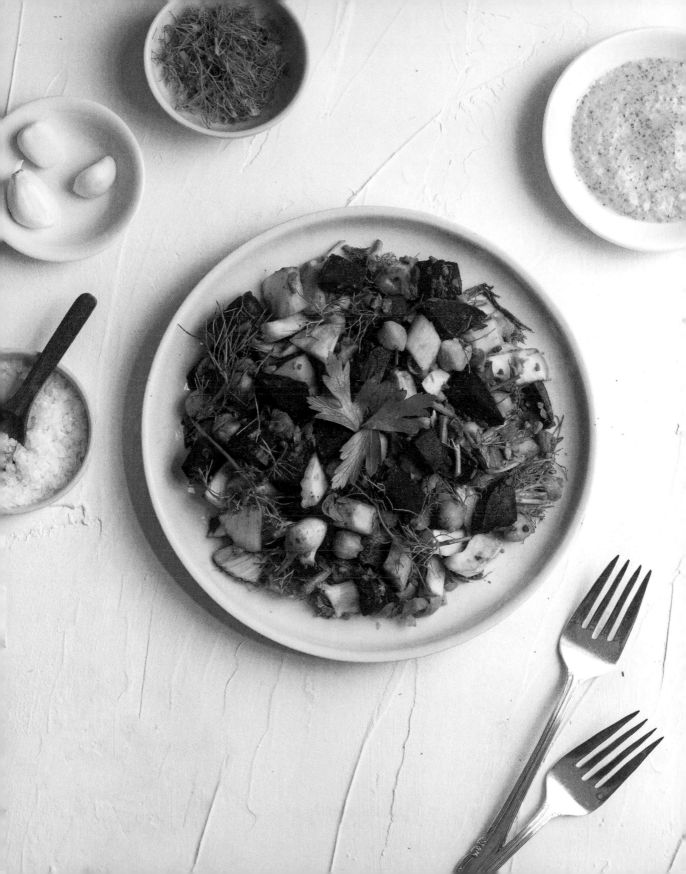

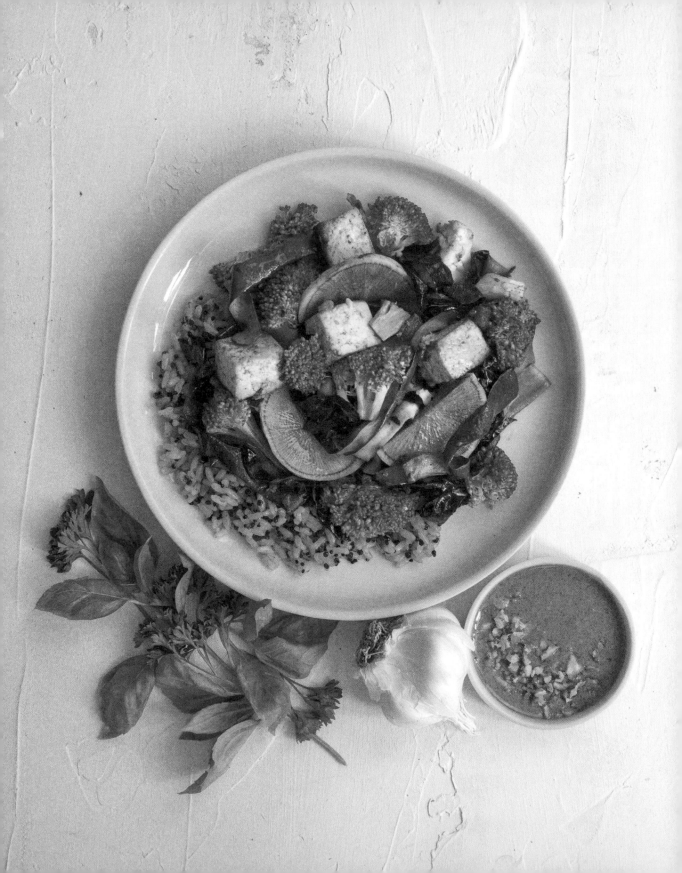

THAI PEANUT STIR-FRY WITH TOFU

PREP TIME: 40 MINUTES   **COOK TIME:** 25 MINUTES   **SERVES** 2

2 to 3 tablespoons Herbal Cooking Oil (page 58)

½ yellow onion, diced

1½ teaspoons grated fresh ginger

½ teaspoon ground turmeric

½ teaspoon ground cumin

½ teaspoon sea salt

½ teaspoon licorice root powder

1 (16-ounce) block extra firm tofu (see Note page 78)

1 garlic clove, minced

½ cup chopped cauliflower

½ cup chopped broccoli

½ cup chopped shredded red cabbage

½ cup chopped zucchini

PEANUT SAUCE

¾ cup natural organic chunky peanut butter

2 tablespoons grated fresh ginger

1 tablespoon white miso paste

1 tablespoon avocado oil

1 tablespoon apple cider vinegar

1 to 2 tablespoons pure maple syrup, to taste

½ teaspoon reishi powder

2 cups cooked brown rice, for serving

2 to 3 slices watermelon radishes, for garnish

Pinch of sesame seeds, for garnish

1 teaspoon diced scallions, for garnish

Nourish yourself by taking the time to prepare a flavorful meal perfectly balanced with savory, spicy, and even sweet flavors. The combination of some of your gut's favorite anti-inflammatory and carminative spices—ginger, turmeric, and cumin—soothes irritation even as it supports strong digestion and absorption of nutrients.

1. Combine the herbal oil, onion, ginger, turmeric, cumin, salt, and licorice root powder in a large sauté pan. Stir to combine, then cook over medium heat for 3 to 5 minutes, until the spices are fragrant and the onion is translucent.

2. Add the tofu and cook, turning it occasionally, for 7 to 10 minutes, until evenly browned and crisp.

3. Add the garlic, cauliflower, broccoli, cabbage, and zucchini, and sauté until the vegetables are tender, 5 to 7 minutes.

4. Make the peanut sauce: Combine the peanut butter, ginger, miso, avocado oil, vinegar, maple syrup, and reishi in a food processor and process until smooth, about 5 minutes (or combine the ingredients in a bowl and whisk vigorously with a fork until smooth). Whisk in hot water 1 tablespoon at a time (about 2 tablespoons total), until the desired consistency is achieved. The sauce should be thick but runny enough to pour.

5. To serve, pile the veggie stir-fry on top of the prepared rice in a bowl. Pour about ¼ cup of the peanut sauce on top of each bowl, garnish with the watermelon radish, sesame seeds, and scallions. Store any extra sauce in an airtight container in the refrigerator for up to 2 weeks.

BAKED APPLES WITH WHIPPED COCONUT CREAM

PREP TIME: 15 MINUTES   **COOK TIME:** 45 MINUTES   **SERVES** 4

⅓ cup gluten-free rolled oats

⅓ cup coconut sugar

½ teaspoon reishi powder

½ teaspoon ground cinnamon

¼ teaspoon ground cloves

¼ teaspoon ground nutmeg

⅛ teaspoon sea salt

1 teaspoon pure vanilla extract, preferably homemade (page 44)

4 apples, cored (see Notes)

2 tablespoons coconut oil, melted

Whipped Coconut Cream with Marshmallow Root (page 49), for garnish (optional)

Imagine the smell of warm cinnamon, cloves, and nutmeg simmered with sweet apple wafting through your house. Now get up and make this recipe! This combination of plants is as warming to the body as it is to the soul. In herbal medicine, cinnamon and cloves are go-to spices to support issues with inflammation. They also provide strong defenses against oxidation—what can happen to cells when they're exposed to unstable free radicals in the environment (think: chemical cleaning products, pollution, stress . . .). Apples are a good source of fiber, adding further digestive wellness. If you don't have (or want to make) the whipped cream, serve with coconut yogurt mixed with a bit of raw honey for an extra microbiome boost. These apples are among the best options for an evening snack, so raise your spoon for more dessert!

1. Preheat the oven to 375°F.

2. Stir together the oats, coconut sugar, reishi, cinnamon, cloves, nutmeg, salt, and vanilla in a small bowl.

3. Tightly pack the oat mixture into each apple core. Place the apples standing upright in a square baking dish.

4. Pour 1 cup water into the bottom of the dish. Loosely cover the dish with aluminum foil and bake for 20 minutes.

5. Remove the foil and spoon 1½ teaspoons of the melted coconut oil over each apple. Bake, uncovered, for another 25 minutes, until the apples are soft and the filling is bubbling.

6. Serve warm, topped with a dollop of whipped coconut cream, if desired. Store leftover apples in an airtight container in the refrigerator for up to 1 day; after that, they will get mushy and considerably less delicious.

NOTES: It is easiest to core the apples using an apple corer tool. You simply need a hollow middle into which you can pack the oat mixture.

Sweet or tart? Everyone has an apple preference. Honeycrisp and Gala are the best options for a sweeter dessert, whereas McIntosh and Granny Smith are more tart.

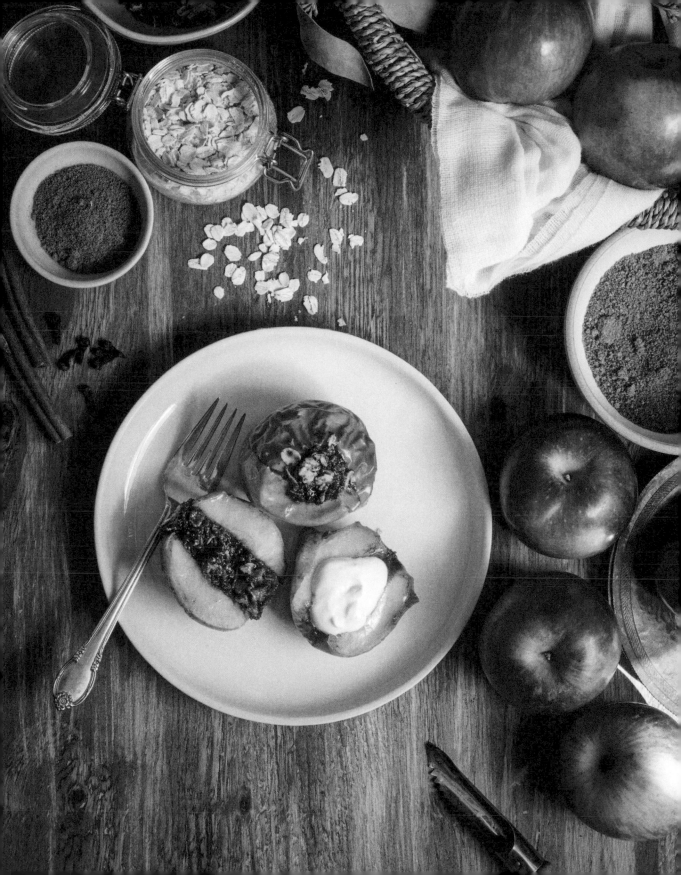

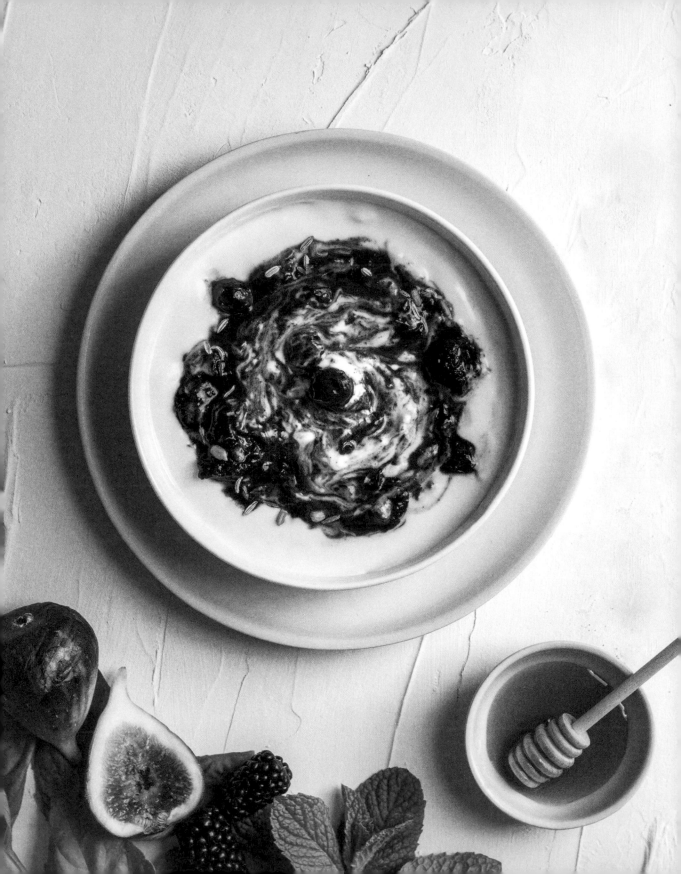

SPICED FIG & BERRY COMPOTE

COOK TIME: 15 MINUTES   **SERVES** 2

1 tablespoon whole fennel seeds

2 tablespoons raw hulled sunflower seeds

1½ teaspoons coconut oil

1 teaspoon grated fresh ginger, or ½ teaspoon ground ginger

½ teaspoon ground cinnamon

½ teaspoon ground nutmeg

¼ teaspoon ground cardamom, or 2 whole green pods

⅛ teaspoon cayenne pepper

½ cup dried or fresh figs, quartered

1½ to 2 cups fresh berries (blueberries, blackberries, and/or raspberries)

½ cup coconut yogurt

1 tablespoon Elderberry Syrup (page 53)

1 teaspoon raw honey

1 teaspoon flaky sea salt

2 tablespoons chopped fresh mint leaves

Frozen treats are at the heart of so many memories and can be the ultimate comfort food for maladies of heart and body. But when it comes to gut-aches (and some heartaches), a pint of you-know-what might do more harm than good, as cold food can (literally) freeze your digestion into a state of shock and extinguish the digestive fire known as *agni* in Ayurveda. This sophisticated dessert meets all the flavor criteria for an indulgent treat and provides the kind of long-term relief your body actually wants when it's crying out for ice cream.

Elderberry syrup is the ultimate natural immune booster, but these potent little berries also soothe digestive cramping and constipation, reduce gas and bloating, and support the detoxifying functions of the liver. Combining gently stimulating spices with probiotic-rich coconut yogurt, this "dessert" can—and should!—be eaten any time of day. Add the compote to a basic grain cereal, any of our Morning-Of Oats recipes (pages 113 to 115), Chia Puddings (page 67), or on top of Vanilla Bean Sweet Potato Banana Pancakes (page 116) for a sweet, delicious morning, afternoon, or evening meal.

1. Toast the fennel and sunflower seeds in a dry medium skillet over low heat until they are fragrant and begin to pop, about 2 minutes. Transfer to a bowl and set aside.

2. In the same pan, stir together the coconut oil, ginger, cinnamon, nutmeg, cardamom, and cayenne, and toast over low heat until the spices are just fragrant, 2 to 3 minutes. Watch this carefully, as the spices can burn quickly.

3. Add the figs and berries and enough water to cover the fruit. Bring to a gentle boil, then reduce the heat to low, simmer, and cook uncovered until the mixture is syrupy, 10 to 12 minutes.

4. Divide the yogurt between two bowls and top each with half the compote. Allow it to melt and swirl together slightly. Sprinkle with the toasted fennel and sunflower seeds.

5. Drizzle the elderberry syrup and honey over the fruit and yogurt, and top with a pinch of salt, the mint leaves, and any additional spices as desired.

SEASONAL EATING

Some people look to the weather to know when the seasons are shifting. But nature also tells us when change is nigh through food. The different kinds of produce available at different times of year tells how we should be eating to deal with the external environment, since nature always gives us what our bodies need.

In our current world, many of us live in different climates from where we grew up, or in places without clear seasons; technology has also allowed for most foods to be available all year long, making it hard to determine what's seasonal. Eating seasonally and locally is one of the many lost arts of our modern diet, and returning to the natural rhythms of the earth's offerings is one way we can reset impaired digestion.

Each individual will have different needs depending on their current state of digestive, mental, and whole-body health, regardless of climate. But one should always prioritize eating what is local/seasonal to where you are at that time. If you live in a temperate region (with seasons), here are some general guidelines for which foods to embrace as you turn the pages of the calendar. While it's common to think of four seasons, Ayurveda bases seasonal eating on the three *growing* seasons, which also may be slightly different based on where you are.

This is not to say you need to deny yourself nonseasonal, nonlocal foods, but rather consider how you can enjoy different fruits and vegetables spread throughout a whole year, rather than a single day. You may pine for blueberries in winter, but can you be okay knowing you can eat your fill of them come summer? When in doubt, turn to your local farmers' market— or your own natural cravings. Notice how seasonal eating affects how you feel in body and mind.

LATE WINTER & SPRING

Alliums: garlic, ramps, spring onion

Cruciferous vegetables

Daikon radish

Grains & legumes: buckwheat, millet, white basmati rice

Light greens: arugula, dandelion, spinach

Raw honey

Spices & herbs: black pepper, burdock, cilantro/coriander, cinnamon, dill, fennel, fenugreek, ground ginger

SUMMER

Aloe

Avacado

Coconut (all forms)

Cucumbers

Eggplant

Fruit

Greens

Plant-based yogurt

Spices & herbs: basil, cardamom, cilantro/coriander, fennel, fresh ginger, mint, oregano, parsley

Tomatoes

Zucchini

FALL & EARLY WINTER

Garlic

Hearty greens: chard, collard greens, kale

Natural sugars: molasses, pure maple syrup

Nuts & seeds (all kinds)

Onion

Root vegetables

Seaweeds

Spices & herbs: black pepper, cardamom, cilantro/coriander, cinnamon, clove, cumin, fennel, fresh ginger, nutmeg, salt

Stewed fruit: apples, dates, figs, pears

Whole grains

CHOCOLATE ALMOND BUTTER OAT BARS

PREP TIME: 10 MINUTES **COOK TIME:** 20 MINUTES **MAKES** 25 BARS

1 tablespoon flax meal

1½ cups gluten-free rolled oats

¼ cup unsweetened applesauce

2 tablespoons almond butter, preferably homemade (page 47)

1 teaspoon pure vanilla extract, preferably homemade (page 44)

¾ cup organic cane sugar

¾ cup almond meal

1 tablespoon ground cinnamon

½ teaspoon baking soda

½ teaspoon sea salt

½ cup chopped dark baking chocolate, nondairy dark chocolate chips, or broken chunks of a dark chocolate bar (70 to 80% cacao) of your choice (2 ounces)

It's natural, and sometimes helpful, to reach back through one's memory to discover the source of digestive trouble. *Was it that week of midnight snacks, that extra cocktail during happy hour, eating lunch at my desk for my whole working life, or that one cookie that turned into a whole box?* Sweets have become the scapegoat of many women's problems and have incurred lots of bad karma among their opponents. But just like any food, sweets in moderation are part of a healthy, balanced relationship between our bodies and what we eat. These bars promise to reverse any bad karma from desserts past, and plant seeds of healing wherever they go—including your belly. With wholesome ingredients and natural sweeteners (it's up to you how sweet you want your chocolate), they'll make you feel happy, satisfied, and loved, which is exactly what all good food does best.

1. Preheat the oven to 350°F. Line an 8-inch square baking pan with reusable parchment, letting the parchment overhang two sides by 2 to 3 inches (so it's easy to lift out bars when they are done).

2. Combine the flax meal with 3 tablespoons hot water in a large bowl and let stand for 5 to 10 minutes, or until thickened.

3. Pulse ¾ cup of the oats in a food processor or spice grinder until it is the consistency of a fine flour.

4. Add the applesauce, almond butter, and vanilla to the bowl with the flax and stir to combine.

5. Add the oat flour and remaining ¾ cup whole oats. Then, one at a time, add the sugar, almond meal, cinnamon, baking soda, and salt, stirring well to mix thoroughly. The batter will be thick and sticky. Fold in the chocolate.

6. Pour the batter into the prepared pan and press it into all the edges to make an even layer. Bake for 20 to 25 minutes, until the top and edges are golden brown. Remove from the oven and let cool completely in the pan. (If you like a cleaner cut, you could put the pan in the refrigerator for 30 to 60 minutes before slicing the bars; but if you don't mind crumbles, you can skip that step.)

7. Using the overhanging parchment, lift the bars from the pan and set them on a cutting board. Cut into 25 squares. Store in an airtight container in the refrigerator for up to 5 days—the bars are very moist and may stick together, so try to place them in as few layers as possible or place a sheet of parchment between layers.

COOKED WATER WITH LEMON

COOK TIME: 10 MINUTES **SERVES** 1

1 to 2 lemon wedges

During the night, our bodies do the incredible work of detoxifying the entire system, rinsing your cells clean of anything that's unneeded from what you took in that day—food or otherwise. Continue that process upon waking by drinking a cup of cooked lemon water. Cooking water makes it easier to digest (since some of the gas evaporates), gives it a smoother taste in the mouth, and prevents the heavy, sloshy feeling some people get after drinking a lot of water. Adding lemon to the water helps fire up the juices in your stomach to prime your digestion for the day and encourages a morning bowel movement that will finish off the nighttime detox process. Try to drink the water all at once in the morning, rather than sipping for hours, to make sure things get moving as soon as possible.

To simplify this part of your morning routine, cut the lemon into wedges at the start of the week and store in the refrigerator so they're ready to go when you wake up. Choose organic lemons whenever possible, especially if you like to let the wedge hang out in your cup.

Consuming cooked water throughout the day is an excellent way to support digestion. Put on a big pot of water in the morning and let it cook while you go about your business (bathing, brushing your teeth, etc.) then drink from the pot all day.

1. Bring a pot of water to a rolling boil over high heat. Reduce to medium heat and continue to boil for 10 minutes, then turn off the heat and let rest, uncovered, while the gases evaporate. You can also boil the water in a tea kettle; just take the top off to allow for evaporation.

2. Pour the water into your favorite mug and squeeze the lemon juice into the water. Sip slowly, without gulping, with limited external stimuli and distractions.

NOTE: If heat is an issue for you, you can alter your Cooked Water a few ways. If you tend toward inflamed digestion, or urgent or loose stools, or are preparing this during the summer, replace the lemon with lime, which is less heating. You also don't need to drink your cooked water hot off the stove—just let the water cool to room temperature, then enjoy.

AYURVEDIC CCF TEA

PREP TIME: 15 MINUTES **SERVES** 1

½ **teaspoon whole cumin seeds**

½ **teaspoon whole coriander seeds**

½ **teaspoon whole fennel seeds**

This combination of seeds is Ayurveda's secret weapon for instant relief from bloating, gas, and indigestion. When combined, their properties provide a balancing effect on the gut to maintain healthy digestion and elimination. Enjoy a small cup before or after a meal, or sip this throughout the day during periods of imbalance. If using ground spices, it may be harder to strain after steeping; that's okay—just know that you might have some residue in your mug. You'll also need a slightly smaller quantity of the ground spices, more like a scant ½ teaspoon. If you need sweetener, add a teaspoon of raw honey to the tea once it's cooled a bit. Ayurveda teaches that cooked honey produces a toxic sludge in the body called *āma*, which is the exact opposite of gut healing!

1. Gently crush all the seeds with a mortar and pestle or between your two hands. Bring 2 cups water to a boil in a small pot. Turn off the heat, then add the seeds. Cover and steep for 5 minutes.

2. Strain the tea through a fine-mesh sieve into a large mug to remove the seeds. You may use the seeds again throughout the day, adding them to a thermos and refreshing them with warm water, leaving the seeds in the water the whole time. You can also make a lighter version of CCF water by simply putting the seeds in warm water and sipping that throughout the day (see Herbal Waters on page 54).

PEPPERMINT LICORICE TEA

PREP TIME: 15 MINUTES   **MAKES** 1 GENEROUS MUG

½ teaspoon dried peppermint

½ teaspoon licorice root

½ teaspoon dried calendula flowers

½ teaspoon dried chamomile flowers

½ teaspoon dried yarrow

1 teaspoon raw honey or other sweetener, or to taste

When you're feeling digestive discomfort, a simple cup of warm tea can be just the right remedy. This collection of herbs is rich in herbal properties specifically suited to relaxing the stomach, releasing gas and cramps, and supporting issues with inflammation. Enjoy this soothing tea to comfort all the senses.

1. Bring 2 cups water to a boil in a tea kettle or small pot.

2. Place the peppermint, licorice root, calendula, chamomile, and yarrow in a tea infuser or reusable tea bag, and put the infuser or tea bag in a mug. Gently pour the boiling water over the herbs. Let steep for 10 minutes.

3. Remove the tea infuser or tea bag. Stir in the honey and enjoy.

LICORICE ROOT *(GLYCYRRHIZA GLABRA)*

NOURISHING HERBS

If you grew up chewing on black licorice candy twists, this potent and beloved herb is for you. Its sweet taste (which is built into its genus name, *Glycyrrhiza*, from the Greek *glykyrrhiza*, which means "sweet") makes it popular among herbalists as a way to balance multi-herb formulas, including in more than five thousand Chinese medicine blends. Licorice is a general tonic with an affinity for the adrenals, anti-inflammatory, mild laxative, antispasmodic, and adaptogen. It's been used for thousands of years all around the world to strengthen the whole body.

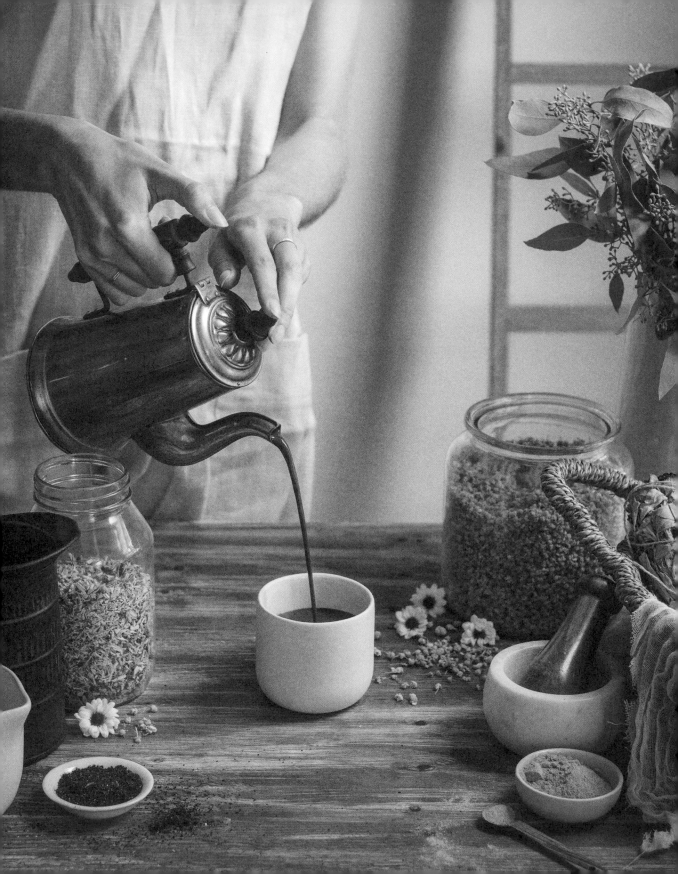

CHICORY ROOT CACAO

PREP TIME: 5 MINUTES   **MAKES** 1 GENEROUS MUG

2 cups almond mylk, preferably homemade (page 43)

1 tablespoon raw cacao powder

1 tablespoon chicory root

1 teaspoon dried chamomile flowers

1 teaspoon licorice root

½ teaspoon ground cardamom

½ teaspoon ground cinnamon

3 whole cloves

1 tablespoon date syrup, or to taste

As is the case for many ingredients in this book, cacao is a true superfood because of all its incredible benefits for the body and mind. We have a different cacao in each section (because: chocolate), but here the main effects are digestive. Raw cacao powder comes from cacao beans that have been fermented, a process that breaks down the bitter tannins in the beans. It's then dried and ground into the powder we can buy and consume. These bitter beans are bursting with antioxidants, which couple beautifully with the prebiotics in chicory and chamomile. All three are bitters, which support digestion and liver function, too. The earthy flavors of this drink are also reminiscent of coffee, making it a perfect substitute for your caffeine habit. While also bitter, coffee tends to overstimulate the nervous system as well as dehydrate the body, thus impeding healthy digestion.

1. Combine the almond mylk, cacao, chicory root, chamomile, licorice root, cardamom, cinnamon, and cloves in a small pan. Bring to a boil over high heat, then reduce the heat to medium, cover, and simmer for 10 minutes. Remove the lid and stir well, then remove from the heat.

2. Strain through a fine-mesh sieve into a mug. Stir in the date syrup, adjusting the sweetness as desired, and enjoy.

NOTE: This cacao is extremely rich and thick, with an intense flavor that will wake you up like the best morning coffee. If you find it too strong, divide it into two servings and dilute it with ½ cup warm water or mylk.

CHICORY ROOT *(CICHORIUM INTYBUS)*

NOURISHING HERBS

Chicory root is a somewhat woody and herbaceous plant of the dandelion family, *Asteraceae*. It has been used as a coffee substitute for centuries, especially in times when coffee was not accessible. It was brought to North America from Europe in the eighteenth century, and the root is the part used in herbal drinks and preparations and can be eaten as a food. Chicory root is a natural source of the prebiotic inulin.

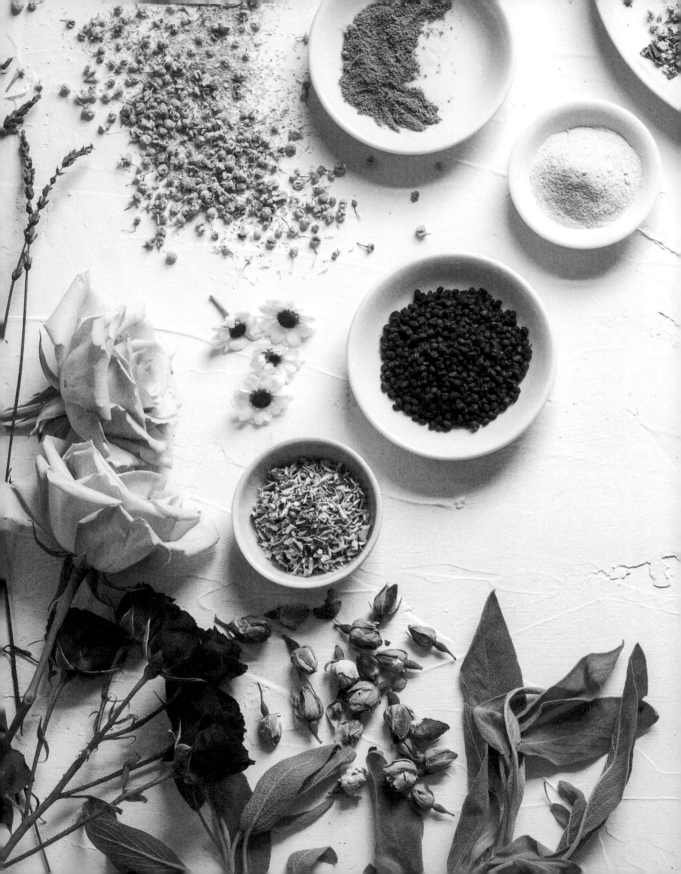

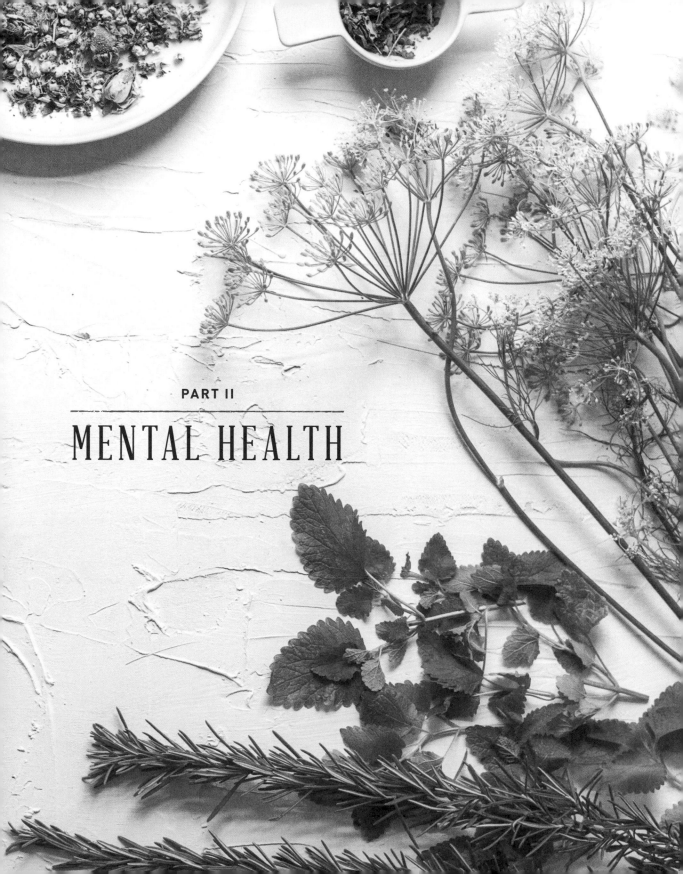

PART II

MENTAL HEALTH

> # Nature quiets the mind
> # by engaging with an intelligence
> # larger than our own.
>
> —TERRY TEMPEST WILLIAMS,
>   "A FEATHER ON PHELPS LAKE"

These words speak to the transition from Part I of this book, on digestion, to Part II, on mental health. We've learned how important proper digestion is to overall health, whether we're digesting food, or emotions, or media. If we're eating but not digesting, the body suffers and can become unwell. Hopefully, the recipes in Part I have helped you find a baseline of digestive balance so that your body is actually absorbing nutrients from the food you're eating, especially the potent nourishment of herbs and spices.

But illness can also stem from a cause that's harder to see, but extremely pervasive, in our modern lives: stress. When we're fielding "urgent" emails 24/7, trying to care for children, doing the work-life-exercise-relationships dance, and eating everything else on our plates, our sympathetic nervous system (fight or flight) flips on to keep us safe from those perceived dangers. You might be familiar with some of the common stress-related symptoms: irregular energy levels and mood, insomnia, fatigue, anxiety and/or depression (they're two sides of the same coin, so if you've felt both, you're not alone!), trouble relating to others, lack of focus, and brain fog, among others. They're the result of our bodies

being flooded with stress hormones needed to help us to run away from the threat at hand—maybe a bear, or our devices—since it's crucial in a moment of real danger to have our blood pumping, our muscles ready to work, and our senses laser-focused.

The thing is, the stress response is only meant to stay on for a short period of time. Yet in our modern world, stress lingers in our bodies far longer than it needs to because of our constant state of stimulation. The longer we remain in a state of stress, the more susceptible we are to getting sick in body, mind, and spirit. Because when the sympathetic nervous system is turned on, its opposite partner, the parasympathetic nervous system—responsible for our bodies' rest and digest functions—gets turned off. The longer we go without digesting what we eat or feel, the fewer nutrients get to our brains, making it hard to maintain balanced thoughts, emotions, and reactions. Go a little longer, and we start to see this cycle penetrate even deeper into our reproductive hormones (which we'll get to in Part III).

Now, the obvious solution to all this is avoiding and eliminating stress. But we can't all relocate to the countryside and grow herbs for the rest of our days—even if we could, we'd have stress there, too! (Anyone who's grown anything knows that bugs or a stretch of lousy weather can make for unhappy times in the garden.) Stress is an inevitable part of being human, and in today's society it's impossible to avoid anxiety altogether. A modest amount of stress, called eustress, is actually good for us, since we need a bit of discomfort, challenge, and urgency in order to get anything done and evolve as individuals. Think about the last time you had to give a presentation or do anything public (social media counts, too)—did you get nervous? Hands a little sweaty? Some butterflies in your belly? That was stress, and a sign that you cared about what you were doing. In fact, the whole reason we wake up in the morning is because our bodies naturally produce a spike in cortisol—the hormone often behind stress-related weight gain. In time, our sources of stress (good or less good) can even become outlets for healing and growth. Still, it's distress (that's the bad kind of stress), or chronic stress, that we need to look out for.

Since we're focusing on food here, it's worth noting that our society creates a decent amount of stress around what and how we eat. Perhaps we're concerned about our bodies looking a certain way, about following the latest fad diets, or even overly concerned with eating healthy. Perhaps an underlying condition associates food with discomfort, and we become hypervigilant out of fear of that potential pain. Perhaps we're so busy we cannot take the time to eat mindfully (see page 72), coupling environmental stress with digestive stress in a negative feedback loop that sucks our immunity and vitality dry.

According to the World Health Organization, one in three people globally suffer from some type of mental illness, but women constitute the majority of these cases, especially when it comes to anxiety, depression, and somatic symptoms (muscle tension, headaches, indigestion, etc.). Depression is twice as common in women as it is in men, and while scientists cannot yet claim a causal relationship between mental health concerns and gender, there are clear correlations when it comes to the increased social, financial, and familial limitations and expectations placed on women in societies around the world. The extra-complicated hormonal dance that women do all month every month also plays a role in these anxiety-related mental health conditions (again, more on that in Part III). The fact that so few people with mental health concerns seek treatment—only two in five—may also have something to do with this gender bias.

Ayurveda teaches that everything can be a poison or a medicine; in other words, the food that might be stressing us out can also be the key to our healing. By eating foods that nurture the gut-brain connection, we can powerfully affect our state of mind about that food, and about everything else. When eating becomes a source of pleasure to all of the senses—its taste, but also its color, aroma, and texture—we have more space to experience pleasure in other parts of our lives. And every bite of relief from the daily grind adds up, so that eventually there's less on our plate that doesn't taste good, and more that does.

In this section, we'll address how anxiety and depression, and their associated symptoms, can be supported by herbs and eating practices. Our intention is to offer you meals that serve as a safe space for feeling and healing—a part of your day where you can trust that what you're eating is working with you, rather than against you, even if the rest of your world feels otherwise. These are foods that are comforting, fragrant, and pretty to look at, designed to share with good company (feeding another pillar of health—connection), and ideal when you're feeling low and want to eat good food with minimal effort. We realize that the notion of cooking at all, let alone with herbs, can be a source of stress for some, so we'll emphasize just how easily herbs can be incorporated into your daily life and ways to be more prepared for potential stressors with a daily routine—including meal prep, make-ahead, and freezer-friendly recipes—so that they're always on hand, and with enough variety to support changes in your mental and physical state.

The herbs in this section fall into many overlapping categories, which you can read more about in the Herbal Actions section on page 26:

+ Adaptogenic
+ Antioxidant
+ Nervine relaxant
+ Sedative
+ Tonic (adrenal, immune, liver, nervous system)

Adaptogens and nervines, which are most common among and within the individual herbs we use in this section (full list on the following page), support the nervous system so the sympathetic and parasympathetic switches don't get turned off and on in extreme ways. Adaptogens are a very special, some might say magical, category of plants that work on the body in nonspecific ways—in other words, they have a unique intelligence to be able to land in the body, find what's imbalanced, and provide whatever support is needed. They're the ultimate stress-busters, but work on the body slowly, accumulating their potency over time, so you won't necessarily see an effect after just one cup of tea. You'll also see more calming herbs than stimulating herbs, though there are recipes that are meant to wake up your system (Spirulina Bliss Smoothie, page 109, and Cayenne Cacao, page 153, are just two examples).

Taken together, the more immediate effects of the nervines and the long-term effects of adaptogens will allow your healing to take place at just the right pace for you. And in that time, you may discover some new truths about yourself, what you like and dislike, and the proper place for your heart to dwell.

It's worth a reminder here that herbal cooking is not meant to be a replacement for medical care. If you or a loved one is suffering, please contact a mental health professional for the support you need to feel well. And if you are currently taking any prescription medications for mental health (or anything), please be sure to consult your doctor before adding medicinal herbs into your diet. While food and herbs can play a huge role in how we feel on all levels, diet is just one part of our beautiful and complex identity, and all parts of us need their own care.

ASHWAGANDHA (*WITHANIA SOMNIFERA*)	adaptogenic, adrenal and nervous system tonic, sedative
ASIAN GINSENG (*PANAX GINSENG*)	adaptogenic, adrenal tonic, sedative
BLACK PEPPER (*PIPER NIGRUM*)	antioxidant
CHAMOMILE (*MATRICARIA RECUTITA*)	nervine relaxant, sedative
LAVENDER (*LAVANDULA ANGUSTIFOLIA*)	nervine relaxant, sedative
LEMON BALM (*MELISSA OFFICINALIS*)	nervine relaxant, sedative
LEMONGRASS (*CYMBOPOGON CITRATUS*)	nervine relaxant
LICORICE ROOT (*GLYCYRRHIZA GLABRA*)	adaptogenic, adrenal and liver tonic
MACA (*LEPIDIUM MEYENII*)	adaptogenic
MUCUNA (*MUCUNA PRURIENS*)	adaptogenic, nervine relaxant, nervous system tonic
OATSTRAW (*AVENA SATIVA*)	demulcent, nervine relaxant, nervous system tonic
PASSIONFLOWER (*PASSIFLORA INCARNATA*)	nervine relaxant, sedative
REISHI (*GANODERMA LUCIDUM*)	adaptogenic, antioxidant, immune tonic
ROSE (*ROSA DAMASCENA*)	nervine relaxant, nervous system tonic
SHIITAKE (*LENTINULA EDODES*)	adaptogenic, immune tonic
SKULLCAP (*SCUTELLARIA LATERIFLORA*)	nervine relaxant, nervous system tonic, sedative
TULSI (*OCIMUM TENUIFLORUM*)	adaptogenic, immune tonic, nervine relaxant
TURMERIC (*CURCUMA LONGA*)	antioxidant, immune and liver tonic

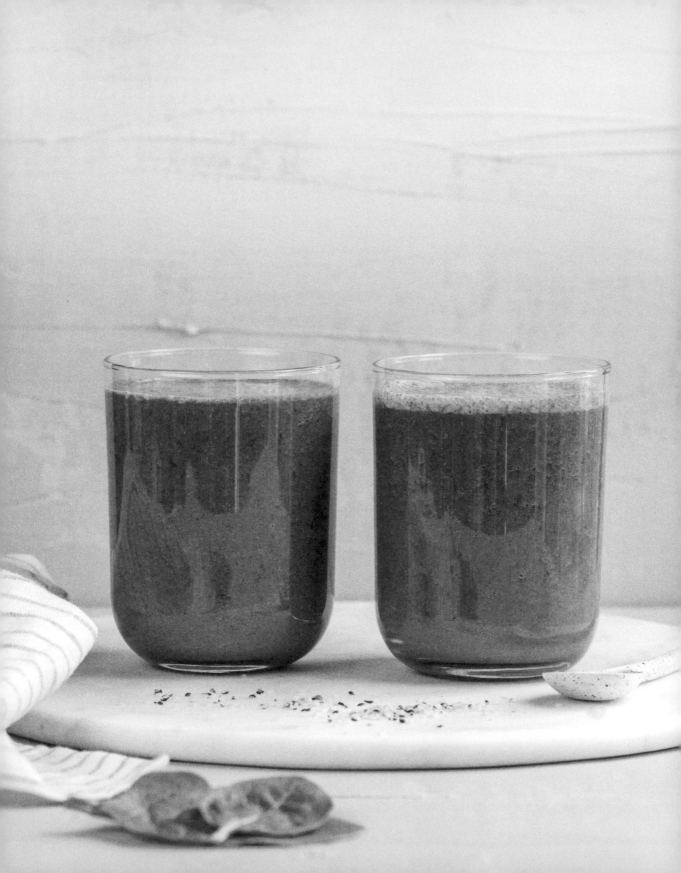

SPIRULINA BLISS SMOOTHIE

PREP TIME: 5 MINUTES   **SERVES** 1

1 cup almond mylk, preferably homemade (page 43)

½ teaspoon plant-based collagen powder

3 tablespoons hemp seeds

2 tablespoons chia seeds

1 tablespoon flax meal

1 tablespoon spirulina powder

½ teaspoon ashwagandha root powder

½ teaspoon Asian ginseng powder

½ cup spinach

½ cup baby kale

1 ripe banana

1 cup ice

Waking up to a forecast of heavy brain fog? This smoothie is formulated with uplifting plants to increase energy and mental stamina, so you can take on the day feeling vibrant and happy. The star is the superfood spirulina, an extremely nutrient-dense bacteria. Because of the potential contamination with toxic strains of algae, be sure to double-check your source of spirulina (we recommend Nutrex Hawaii). Also keep in mind that as a superfood, spirulina is extremely expensive to produce, financially and environmentally. It's not meant to be used as a substitute for nutrition found in whole foods. Enjoy it when your body or mood needs a small boost.

Combine the mylk, collagen, hemp seeds, chia seeds, flax meal, spirulina, ashwagandha, and ginseng in a high-speed blender. Add the spinach, kale, banana, and ice. Blend on high for 1 minute, or until smooth. Pour into a glass and serve immediately.

ASHWAGANDHA *(WITHANIA SOMNIFERA)*

NOURISHING HERBS

Named after its unusual odor (the word *ashwagandha* means "the smell and strength of a horse" in Sanskrit), and known as Indian ginseng and winter cherry, ashwagandha is a prized member of the Ayurvedic pharmacopeia for its adaptogenic properties, which means it has the ability to support the whole system in a number of ways: as a stimulant that boosts memory, vitality, and endurance, or as a relaxant that promotes sleep and grounding. It's also a potent aphrodisiac with an affinity to the male reproductive system, though all genders can benefit from its use. Typically it is taken as part of a warm milk tonic with honey and a pinch of cinnamon or nutmeg, and is more commonly consumed during the fall and winter months, as it has heating properties.

BLUEBERRY, ROSE & WALNUT GRANOLA

PREP TIME: 10 MINUTES   **COOK TIME:** 20 MINUTES   **MAKES** 8 CUPS

2 tablespoons flax meal

2 cups gluten-free rolled oats

1 cup quinoa flakes

⅔ cup raw walnuts, chopped

¼ cup raw hulled sunflower seeds

¼ cup unsweetened coconut chips

1½ tablespoons mucuna powder

1 tablespoon gelatinized maca powder (see Note)

2 teaspoons ground cinnamon

1 teaspoon flaky sea salt

½ teaspoon ground ginger

½ cup pure maple syrup

¼ cup coconut oil, melted

2 teaspoons pure vanilla extract, preferably homemade (page 44)

⅔ cup dried blueberries

⅓ cup goji berries

3 tablespoons lightly crushed dried culinary-grade rose petals (see Note)

We take in our food with the totality of our five senses, which is why it's so important to choose foods that satisfy us by sight, smell, sound, and texture, as well as taste. This clumpy-crunchy granola checks all the boxes with its vibrant hues and dreamy aroma that will summon you out of bed and to the breakfast table even on the dreariest of days. Herbal support comes from *Mucuna pruriens*, or velvet bean, a plant that has been used in Ayurveda and Chinese medicine for centuries as a natural mood-booster. Mucuna contains dopamine-activating amino acids, protects against neurological disorders, enhances virility, and acts as an antioxidant. Maca, also known as Peruvian ginseng, is similarly revered in South America as a superfood, aphrodisiac, and endurance- and mood-enhancer. Just a few spoonfuls of this granola in the morning, or any time of day, can help you find the headspace to stop and smell the roses, whether you're strolling in a garden or sitting down for a meal.

---

1. Preheat the oven to 400°F. Line a large baking sheet with reusable parchment.

2. Stir together the flax meal and 6 tablespoons hot water into a large bowl and let stand for 5 minutes, or until thickened.

3. Add the oats, quinoa flakes, walnuts, sunflower seeds, coconut chips, mucuna, maca, cinnamon, salt, and ginger to the bowl with the flax. Stir to combine, then add the maple syrup, coconut oil, and vanilla. Mix well.

4. Spread the granola evenly over the prepared baking sheet and bake for 20 minutes, or until just browned. Let cool completely before adding the blueberries, goji berries, and rose petals. You can do this by gently tossing the ingredients on the baking sheet, or by putting the granola, fruit, and petals in a large jar (or two) and shaking to combine. Store in the freezer or refrigerator (to maintain the granola's crunch) for up to 3 months.

NOTE: We recommend gelatinized maca powder rather than raw. This processing of the plant makes it easier to digest for most, and therefore more supportive to the entire system.

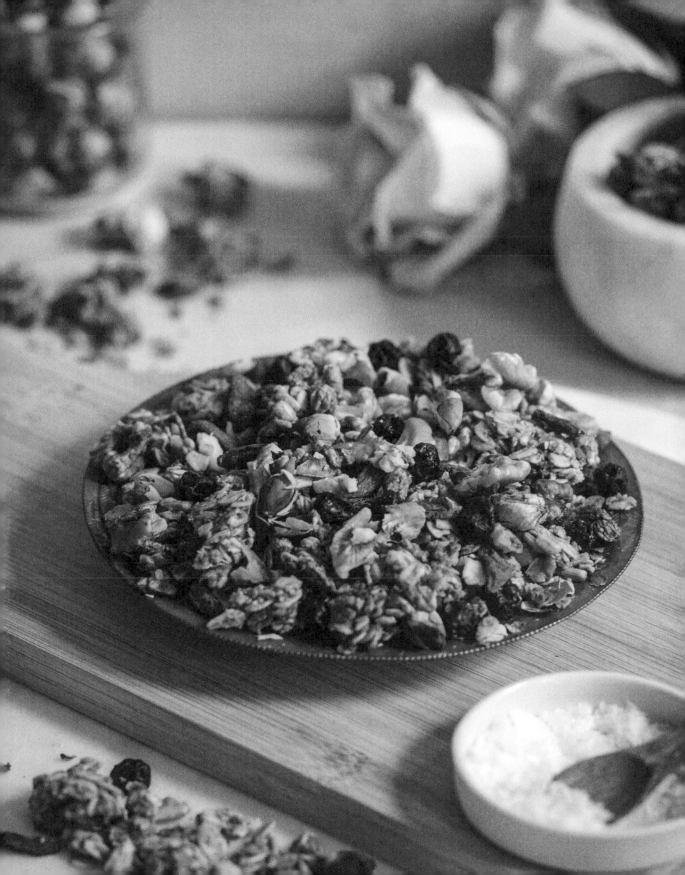

GRATITUDE REFLECTION

HONORING THE ROOTS OF OUR MEAL

Whenever we eat, we're not just taking in isolated nutrients—carbs, proteins, fats, vitamins, minerals, etc. We're taking in the whole story of our food, from the soil in which it was grown to the people who harvested it and all the hands and places it passed through to get to us. Take a moment to reflect on those human and non-human nutrients within your meal before your first bite. Visualize the place where your food came from and the faces of the people involved in its journey. Silently thank the land and those individuals for supplying the ingredients for your meal. In doing so, your mind and body will be primed to digest your food under conditions of gratitude and connection.

MORNING-OF OATS

Overnight oats can change your life, or at least your breakfast. But when you wake up and realize you *forgot* to prep your oats, suddenly your breakfast dream becomes a nightmare. No matter what prevented you from getting ahead of tomorrow's meals, this morning-of solution takes all the anxiety out of preparing a breakfast that's hearty, comforting, and warm (i.e., easier on your gut) at the start of your day.

If you're taking your meal to-go, you can mix it up right in a thermos container and have your oats perfectly cooked by the time you land at your desk. Or if you're at home, you can let them cook while you shower, meditate, or cuddle with a furry friend (animal or human). Be sure to mix together the dry ingredients before you add the water to ensure an even consistency once it's set. The general ratio of 1 part oats to 2 parts water works well with most add-ins, but if you're using more powders or won't be eating the oatmeal for a while, you may need to refresh it with a bit more water when you're ready to eat. Believe it or not, this method of soaking the oats in hot water makes them even creamier than cooking them on the stovetop.

These combos make use of sweet or savory ingredients, which will keep you from getting bored by your breakfast throughout your week. Once you've mastered the technique and learn what add-ins serve you best, feel free to experiment with other combinations.

PB&E (PEANUT BUTTER & ELDERBERRY)

PREP TIME: 10 MINUTES **SERVES** 1

⅓ cup gluten-free
   rolled oats

1 tablespoon peanut
   butter

½ teaspoon
   ashwagandha
   root powder

⅔ cup boiling water

2 teaspoons Elderberry
   Syrup (page 53)

1 tablespoon chia seeds

This isn't your average PB&J—immune-boosting elderberry and adaptogenic ashwagandha infuse these oats with support for your whole body.

Stir together the oats, peanut butter, and ashwagandha in a bowl or carry container. Add the boiling water, stir, and let sit for 10 minutes, or until the oats have absorbed the water. Drizzle with the elderberry syrup and sprinkle the chia seeds on top.

CHERRY VANILLA

PREP TIME: 10 MINUTES   **SERVES** 1

⅓ cup gluten-free rolled oats

⅓ cup dried cherries

1 teaspoon ground cinnamon

1 teaspoon gelatinized maca powder

½ teaspoon ground cardamom

½ teaspoon pure vanilla extract, preferably homemade (page 44)

⅔ cup boiling water

1 tablespoon coconut oil, melted, or tahini, preferably homemade (page 47)

Sweet and sour, fruity and fragrant, these oats bring brightness to your tongue and morning. Use coconut oil for a bit of creaminess in the warmer months, or tahini in the cooler months.

Stir together the oats, cherries, cinnamon, maca, cardamom, and vanilla in a bowl or carry container. Add the boiling water, stir, and let sit for 10 minutes, or until the oats have absorbed the water. Drizzle with the coconut oil.

NUTS FOR NUTS

PREP TIME: 10 MINUTES   **SERVES** 1

⅓ cup gluten-free rolled oats

3 tablespoons unsweetened coconut flakes or chips

2 tablespoons chopped raw walnuts

2 tablespoons chopped raw hazelnuts

2 teaspoons ground cinnamon

⅔ cup boiling water

1 teaspoon pure maple syrup

Full of texture and grounding fats, this nutty mix is the ultimate brain food, especially when you're feeling a bit . . . nuts!

Stir together the oats, coconut, walnuts, hazelnuts, and cinnamon in a bowl or carry container. Add the boiling water, stir, and let sit for 10 minutes, or until the oats have absorbed the water. Drizzle with the maple syrup.

MIGHTY MISO MUSHROOM

PREP TIME: 12 MINUTES   **SERVES** 1

2 tablespoons white
  or red miso paste

¾ cup plus
  2 tablespoons
  boiling water

⅓ cup gluten-free
  rolled oats

¼ cup dried mushrooms

½ sheet kombu, broken
  into small pieces

1 teaspoon ground
  ginger

1 cup packed greens,
  such as spinach
  or Swiss chard
  (leaves only)

Umami flavor for breakfast, plus fiber-rich greens to keep you full until lunch.

Whisk together the miso and 2 tablespoons of the boiling water in a bowl or carry container until smooth. Add the oats, mushrooms, kombu, and ginger; stir to combine with the miso. Place the greens on top, then pour in the remaining ¾ cup boiling water, stir, and let sit for 10 minutes, or until the oats have absorbed the water and the greens have wilted.

SCRAMBLED PLANTS

PREP TIME: 10 MINUTES   **SERVES** 1

⅓ cup gluten-free
  rolled oats

2 tablespoons
  nutritional yeast

1 tablespoon flax meal

½ teaspoon paprika

½ teaspoon ground
  turmeric

¼ teaspoon Umami
  Spice Blend (page 50)

1 cup boiling water

Pinch of freshly ground
  black pepper

Pinch of black salt

Optional toppings:
  avocado slices,
  chopped fresh
  parsley, cilantro,
  or basil leaves

Move over, tofu, oats are the new plant-based scramble.

Stir together the oats, nutritional yeast, flax meal, paprika, turmeric, and spice blend in a bowl or carry container. Pour the boiling water over the mixture, stir, and let stand for 10 minutes, or until the oats have absorbed the water. Season with the pepper and black salt, then add your toppings, if desired. (If you're taking this on the go, store the toppings in a separate container from the oatmeal until you're ready to eat.)

VANILLA BEAN SWEET POTATO BANANA PANCAKES

PREP TIME: 10 MINUTES   **COOK TIME:** 20 MINUTES   **MAKES** 10 PANCAKES

½ cup peeled baked sweet potato

1 ripe medium banana

½ cup gluten-free rolled oats

½ cup gluten-free measure-for-measure flour blend

1 tablespoon gelatinized maca powder

1 tablespoon chia seeds

1¼ cups almond mylk, preferably homemade (page 43)

½ teaspoon pure vanilla extract, preferably homemade (page 44)

1 teaspoon ground cinnamon

½ teaspoon ground nutmeg

Pinch of sea salt

1 tablespoon baking powder

Nonstick cooking spray or coconut oil

Optional toppings: drizzle of tahini or almond butter (preferably homemade, page 47), raw honey or pure maple syrup, jelly or Elderberry Syrup (page 53)

Nothing says "comfort" quite like sitting down in front of a plate of pancakes. From the aroma to the texture, this classic breakfast tastes like those lazy weekends when you stay in your pajamas all day and practice the art of doing less. The natural sources of sweetness in these pancakes—sweet potato and banana—help you feel rooted and deeply satiated, as well as nourished with important vitamins and minerals. Vanilla may seem like a humble pantry staple, but it's actually an ancient superfood with powerful effects on mood, thanks to its comforting scent. Don't reserve your pancakes for the weekend—when you make a whole batch on Sunday, you'll have plenty left over for breakfast throughout the week, or really any time of day when you're looking for a healthy nosh (assuming there are any left!).

1. Combine the sweet potato and banana in a medium bowl and mash together with a fork, potato masher, or hand mixer. (It doesn't need to be perfectly smooth at this stage, but work to break up the big chunks.)

2. Add the oats, flour blend, maca, and chia. Stir to combine.

3. Add the mylk, vanilla, cinnamon, nutmeg, and salt; stir well. At this stage, the batter should be thick but loose enough to pour easily; stir in more liquid, a little at a time, if the batter is too thick or more oats if it is too thin. The banana and sweet potato should also be smooth and fully mashed. Add the baking powder and stir to incorporate.

4. Lightly coat a large skillet with cooking spray and set it over low heat. Using a quarter-cup measuring cup, scoop out some batter and pour it in an even layer onto the skillet. Repeat to fit as many pancakes as your skillet will hold without crowding them. Cook until bubbles appear on the tops of the pancakes and the bottoms are firm when you peek underneath with a spatula. Flip and cook until golden brown and crispy on both sides. (The insides might be slightly soft, but think of cookies that are moist in the center and crisp on the outside—yum!) Transfer the pancakes to a dish, cover with foil or a tea towel to keep warm, and repeat with the remaining batter. Serve warm, with the toppings of your choice.

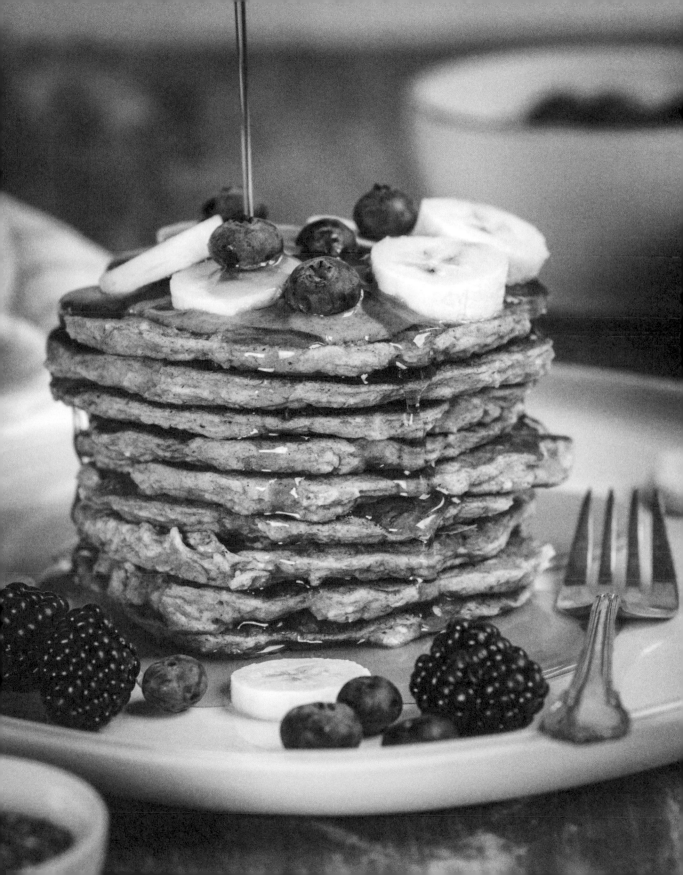

ENERGIZING SUN SALUTATIONS

Invigorating the body and the breath can help to uplift your spirits during periods of low mood or fatigue. Take 10 minutes to incorporate these sun salutations into your morning routine, or as a break in the afternoon when the 3 p.m. slump hits.

STAND tall with your feet under your hips. Set your gaze at the horizon line in front of you, but soften your eyes as if you could see to the far sides of the space you're standing in.

BREATHE IN, and sweep your arms out to the sides and up, touching your palms overhead and following your hands with your eyes as you do so. Stretch long from your heels to your hands, as if you could lengthen the space between your ribs.

BREATHE OUT, and bring your hands through the midline of your body and bow over your legs into a forward fold; bend your knees if the backs of your legs are tight. Inhale again and step, one foot at a time, backward into a Downward Facing Dog posture, making a triangle shape with your body (hands and feet the bottom points, hips the top point). Exhale fully in dog pose.

LOOK forward to your hands with your next inhale, and soften your knees. Exhale, and step your feet to the top of your space, between your hands.

SWEEP your arms out the side and up as you inhale and rise to stand upright. With your exhalation, bring your hands to prayer at your sternum, looking forward with open eyes.

COMPLETE 4 to 6 rounds, switching which foot you step back with first each time.

You can also practice the salutations seated, using your arms only. Simply sweep your arms up and look at your hands in a prayer above your head with an inhalation; then exhale and bring your hands to your heart. Keep your eyes open, following your hands with your gaze. Complete 6 to 10 rounds.

GINSENG CILANTRO LIME CAULIFLOWER RICE

PREP TIME: 15 MINUTES   **COOK TIME:** 25 MINUTES   **SERVES** 2

- 4 to 5 cups fresh cauliflower florets
- 2 tablespoons white hulled sesame seeds
- 2 tablespoons coconut oil
- ½ cup chopped scallions, plus more for garnish
- 1 (1-inch) piece fresh ginger, coarsely chopped
- 3 teaspoons tamari
- 1 tablespoon rice vinegar
- 1 teaspoon white miso paste
- 1 teaspoon Asian ginseng powder
- Zest and juice of 1 lime
- Handful of fresh cilantro, chopped, for garnish

While we're big fans of regular rice here—no carb shame!—cauliflower rice is a lovely alternative and makes a lighter, more energizing base, especially when your energy or mood level is low. By "frying" with coconut oil, you get a dose of brain food as well, and the ginseng, ginger, lime, and miso give you a big zing of flavor and herbal support. This dish tastes like the definition of umami—or maybe like peace.

1. Working in small batches, pulse the cauliflower florets in a food processor or blender until broken down to resemble rice in size. Set aside.

2. Toast the sesame seeds in a dry large skillet over medium-low heat until brown and fragrant, about 1 minute. Set aside.

3. In the same skillet, melt the coconut oil over medium heat. Add the scallions and ginger. Cook for about 1 minute, until the scallions begin to soften. Add the cauliflower and stir to coat evenly in the oil. Add 1 teaspoon of the tamari; stir to coat. Cook over high heat for 15 to 20 minutes, until the cauliflower begins to brown slightly. (It won't "fry" all the way like real rice does.)

4. Meanwhile, whisk together the remaining 2 teaspoons of tamari, the vinegar, miso, ginseng, and lime zest and juice in a small bowl.

5. To serve, divide the cauliflower among two bowls. Pour the sauce evenly over the cauliflower, then top with the toasted sesame seeds, additional scallions, a squeeze of lime juice, and the cilantro.

LEAFY GREENS SALAD WITH WALNUTS & BERRIES

PREP TIME: 10 MINUTES **SERVES** 2

2 cups mixed tender greens, such as arugula, spinach, and butter lettuce

1 tablespoon Herbal Cooking Oil (page 58)

1 tablespoon fresh lemon juice

Sea salt and freshly ground black pepper

2 cups cubed watermelon

1 cup quartered fresh strawberries

½ cup fresh blueberries

½ cup finely chopped cucumber

¼ cup chopped raw walnuts

4 mint leaves, finely chopped

¼ cup Herbal Balsamic Vinegar (page 56)

Most of the recipes in this book are cooked and served warm, for the purpose of enhancing digestibility. But when the time is right—in this case, summer—the juicy, bright, and refreshing flavors of fruit, cucumber, greens, and mint make for a mouthful of joy (see the section on Seasonal Eating on page 94 for more). The crunch of walnuts on top also boosts brain health with their good-for-you fats. Due to the delicate nature of the greens, it's best to eat this as soon as it's prepared; if you need to pack it for some reason, store the salad and dressing in separate containers.

1. Place the greens in a bowl or on a plate and toss with the herbal cooking oil and lemon juice. Season with salt and pepper.

2. Top with the watermelon, strawberries, blueberries, cucumber, walnuts, and mint and lightly toss. Drizzle with the vinegar and serve immediately.

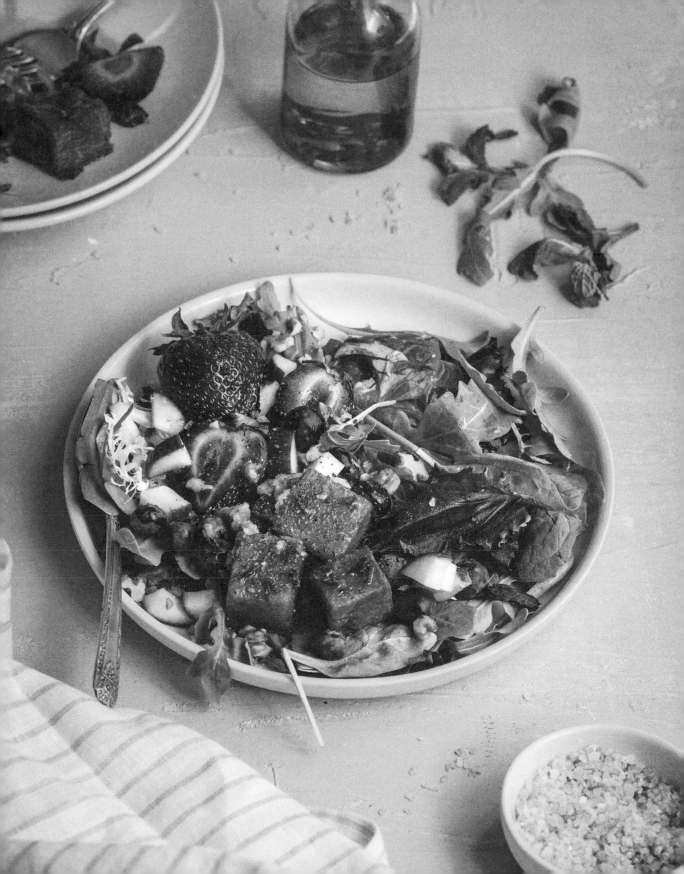

HEARTWARMING VEGAN CHILI

PREP TIME: 10 MINUTES, PLUS OVERNIGHT SOAKING   **COOK TIME:** 50 MINUTES   **SERVES** 6

1 tablespoon avocado oil

1 small onion, chopped

3 or 4 small sweet potatoes, cubed

1 tablespoon dried basil

1 teaspoon sea salt

½ teaspoon freshly ground black pepper

4 cups vegetable broth

2 cups tomato sauce

¼ cup white cooking wine

½ cup dried kidney beans, soaked overnight, or 1 cup canned kidney beans, drained and rinsed

½ cup dried lentils

2 cups frozen vegetable blend (such as peas, carrots, corn, and green beans)

1 cup fresh spinach

Toppings of your choice, such as fresh parsley or Plant Parmesan (page 50), for serving

Gluten-free or sourdough bread (see page 130), for serving

Nature doesn't feel the need to confuse us too much. For the most part, what you see is what you get—and what you see in this bowl of chili is no exception. Heart-shaped legumes, chunks of grounding root vegetables, and aromatic greens and herbs reflect the way this recipe nourishes the spirit as much as the body. While the spices are on the lighter side, they give enough heat to enliven every bite, while the main ingredients ground and restore. The flavor develops more over time, making this an ideal recipe to cook a big batch of for a few days' worth of meals, but it's also quick enough to pull together even on the busiest night.

1. Heat the avocado oil in a heavy-bottomed pot over medium heat. Add the onion and sweet potatoes. Cook for 3 to 4 minutes, until fragrant. Stir in the basil, salt, and pepper.

2. Pour in the broth, tomato sauce, wine, kidney beans (if using dried beans), lentils, and frozen veggies. Bring the mixture to a boil, then reduce the heat to low, cover, and simmer for 35 to 40 minutes, until the legumes are soft.

3. Uncover and stir in the spinach (and the kidney beans, if using canned beans). Cook until the spinach is wilted and everything is warmed through, 3 to 5 minutes. Serve warm, with your favorite toppings or bread. Store leftovers in an airtight container in the refrigerator for up to 1 week in the freezer for up to 3 months.

LOADED BAKED SWEET POTATOES

PREP TIME: 5 MINUTES   **COOK TIME:** 1 HOUR   **SERVES** 2 AS A MAIN, 4 AS A SIDE

2 medium sweet potatoes

OPTIONAL TOPPINGS
Drizzle avocado oil

½ medium onion, diced

½ cup cooked or canned black beans (page 51), drained and rinsed

½ cup corn kernels

¼ cup Savory Cashew Cream (page 48)

½ cup Heartwarming Vegan Chili (page 122)

1 tablespoon chopped fresh parsley leaves

1 tablespoon chopped fresh cilantro, leaves and stems

1 tablespoon Plant Parmesan (page 50)

Sea salt and freshly ground black pepper

Entire populations in Papua New Guinea eat a diet of almost exclusively sweet potatoes and have remarkable health. Now, we're not suggesting anything as drastic as a sweet potato diet, but you might want to embrace this naturally sweet, satisfying, and nutritionally complete food more often. These loaded baked sweet potatoes are a great meal to make for a crowd, so you can spread the sweet potato wealth—and experience those moments of connection that are essential to mental wellness. (Remember, it's one of the pillars of health!) Simply adjust the quantities of the ingredients and feel free to add your own favorites to the topping menu for a personalized potato bar.

---

1. Preheat the oven to 400°F. Line a baking sheet with a silicone baking mat or reusable parchment.

2. Wash the sweet potatoes and poke holes on each side with a fork. Bake for 1 hour, or until tender.

3. Remove the sweet potatoes from the oven, cut each in half, drizzle with the avocado oil, and have fun topping!

LEMONGRASS SPRING ROLLS WITH TEMPEH

PREP TIME: 30 MINUTES   **COOK TIME:** 20 MINUTES   **MAKES** 4 SPRING ROLLS

MARINATED TEMPEH
1 lemongrass stalk

8 ounces tempeh, cut into ½-inch-thick slices

1 garlic clove, peeled

½ cup coconut aminos

¼ cup apple cider vinegar

SPRING ROLLS
8 rice paper wrappers

1 mango, peeled and cut into matchsticks

½ red bell pepper, cut into matchsticks

¼ cup cucumber, cut into matchsticks

1 small bunch green-leaf lettuce

Leaves from 1 small bunch basil (about 12)

Peanut Sauce (page 89), for dipping

While the ingredients of these spring rolls nourish our bodies, it's important to notice their uplifting effects on your mood, as well. Lemongrass releases a fragrance that helps us feel cheery, even as it provides a sense of calm and well-being, due to its nervine and relaxant herbal properties. The process of making the rolls is a practice of mindfulness in and of itself, giving the entire meal from start to finish a zen, yet invigorating, vibe.

1. Make the marinated tempeh: Preheat the oven to 375°F. Line a baking sheet with reusable parchment.

2. Remove the tough outer layers of the lemongrass stalk and cut off the bottom bulb. Trim off and discard the tougher top portion of the stalk, leaving just the softer white bottom. Mince the lemongrass and transfer to a food processor.

3. Add the garlic, coconut aminos, and vinegar and process on high until smooth.

4. Arrange the sliced tempeh in a single layer in a wide shallow bowl or a rectangular container. Pour the lemongrass marinade over the tempeh. Flip the tempeh until all the slices are thoroughly coated. Set aside to marinate for 20 minutes, flipping the tempeh two or three times to coat in the marinade.

5. Place the marinated tempeh in a single layer on the prepared baking sheet, reserving the marinade remaining in the container. Bake the tempeh for 10 minutes, then flip and bake for another 10 minutes. Remove from the oven and let cool on the pan.

6. Make the spring rolls: Fill a large shallow bowl with warm water, about ½ inch deep. Quickly dip 2 rice paper wrappers in the water just to wet. Remove them, letting the excess water drip off, then lay them flat on a clean work surface with a slight overlap (think of a Venn diagram with a very large middle overlapped section).

7. Place 2 or 3 slices of mango, bell pepper, and cucumber in the center of the wrapper. Add 1 leaf of lettuce and 3 or 4 basil leaves, then top with a slice of tempeh. Make sure to keep 1 to 2 inches of the wrapper uncovered around the edges so they can be folded in. Gently pull the bottom edge of the wrapper up and tuck it over the filling, rolling away from you. Next, fold in the sides so the filling is enclosed. Continue to roll the wrapper away from you, pulling and tucking tightly until it is completely rolled. Place the spring roll on a plate and repeat to assemble the remaining rolls.

8. Serve with peanut sauce for dipping.

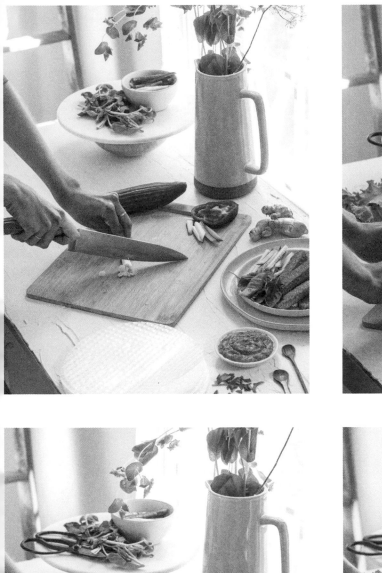
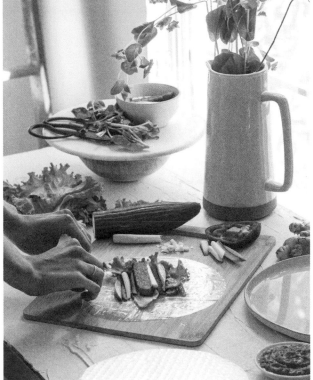
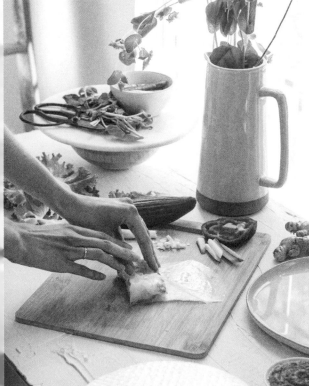
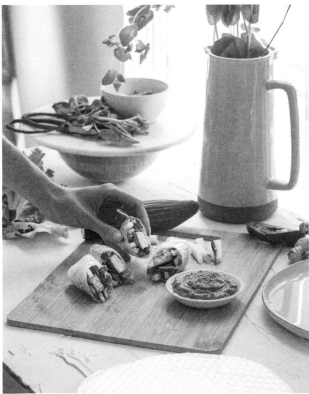

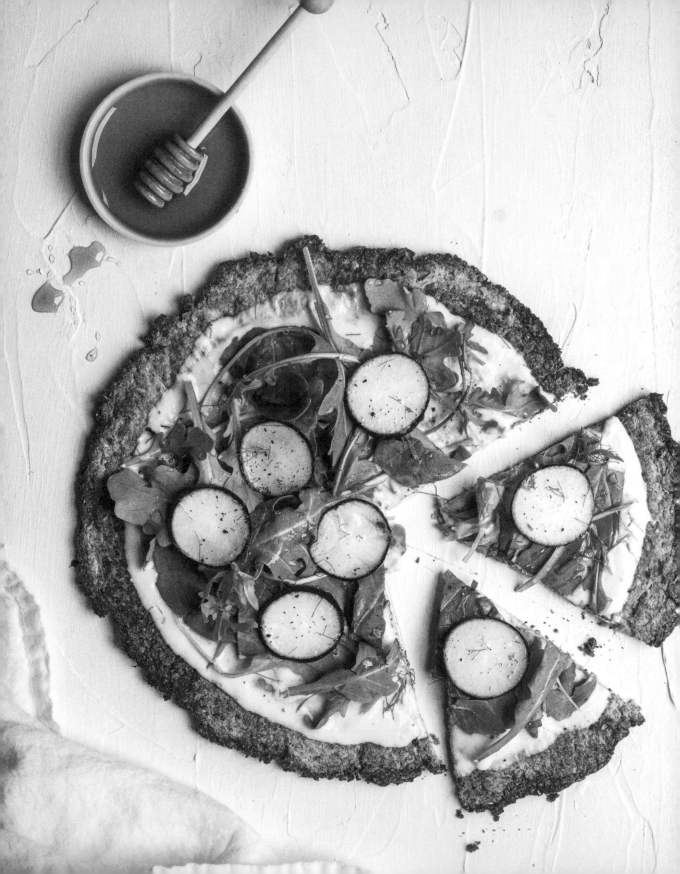

CAULIFLOWER PIZZA WITH CASHEW CREAM, FENNEL, ARUGULA & HONEY

PREP TIME: 30 MINUTES   **COOK TIME:** 45 MINUTES   **MAKES** 1 12- TO 14-INCH PIZZA, TO SERVE 3 TO 4

1½ pounds fresh cauliflower florets

½ cup almond flour

3 tablespoons flax meal

½ teaspoon sea salt

½ teaspoon garlic powder

1 teaspoon ashwagandha root powder

½ teaspoon dried oregano

1 cup Cashew Cream (Plain or Savory, page 48)

½ cup arugula

2 tablespoons fresh fennel bulb, chopped

¼ cup radishes, thinly sliced

Raw honey, for drizzling

Pizza is one of the ultimate connection foods—it's basically designed to be shared, pulled apart, and eaten with both hands and faces full of smiles. This is a more wholesome take on your classic take-out, with toppings that will support healthy digestion by feeding your gut, in addition to feeding your relationships. Ashwagandha adds an adaptogenic kick to the unique cauliflower crust, baking grounding and rejuvenating energy right into every slice of your pizza.

1. Preheat the oven to 400°F. Line a large baking sheet with reusable parchment.

2. Fill a large pot with 3 to 4 cups water and place a steamer basket inside (the water should not come above the bottom of the basket). Put the cauliflower in the basket and bring the water to a boil. Cover the pot and reduce the heat to medium-low. Steam the cauliflower until it is extremely tender, about 15 minutes. Drain and transfer to a food processor. Process on high until the cauliflower resembles grains of rice. Let cool, about 5 minutes.

3. Transfer the cauliflower rice to the center of a clean thin dish towel or a nut-milk bag. Squeeze until all the excess moisture is removed from the cauliflower. (There will be about ½ cup of liquid pressed out.) Put the drained cauliflower in a large bowl, then add the almond flour, flax meal, salt, garlic powder, ashwagandha, and oregano. Stir well to combine, using your hands if needed so it sticks together.

4. Use your hands to shape the crust into an even round, 12 to 14 inches in diameter, onto the prepared baking sheet. The thinner and flatter the crust, the better.

5. Bake the crust for 30 minutes. Remove from the oven and carefully loosen the parchment from the crust. Wearing oven mitts, place one hand below the crust and one hand on top to lift and flip it. Return it to the oven for another 10 to 15 minutes, until golden and dry to the touch.

6. Spread the cashew cream over the crust and top with the arugula, fennel, radishes, and any other desired toppings (the options are endless!). Drizzle with honey, slice, and serve.

SPAGHETTI SQUASH BOATS WITH BASIL & OREGANO

PREP TIME: 10 MINUTES   **COOK TIME:** 1 HOUR   **SERVES** 2

1 medium spaghetti squash

½ (16-ounce) block firm tofu, pressed (see Note page 78)

½ cup diced onion

2 cups chopped fresh tomatoes

¼ cup tomato purée

¼ cup chopped fresh basil, plus more for garnish

¼ cup chopped fresh oregano, plus more for garnish

1½ tablespoons nutritional yeast

3 cups chopped fresh spinach

Sea salt and freshly ground black pepper

Plant Parmesan (page 50), for garnish (optional)

Italians know how to live well: whether it's the wine, the olive oil, or the big personalities cooking and serving it all, an Italian meal is almost always guaranteed to result in satisfaction. If traditional Italian dishes don't quite work with your dietary needs (ahem, vegan and gluten-free), you can still savor the taste, aroma, and colors of this nourishing cuisine—the herbal way. These spaghetti squash boats feed your body and mind with pungent herbs, iron-rich spinach, and a boost of vitamin B12 (an essential vitamin, especially for vegans) from the nutritional yeast for your brain. Enjoy this filling, aromatic, minimal waste (it comes with its own bowl!) meal with your partner, roommate, or best friend, add a loaf of (gluten-free) sourdough bread, and watch your dinner turn into a late-night feelings fest—and a meal to remember.

1. Preheat the oven to 400°F. Line a rimmed baking sheet with reusable parchment.

2. Cut the squash in half lengthwise. Place the halves cut-side down on the prepared baking sheet and pour ½ cup water onto the pan. Roast for 45 minutes to 1 hour, depending on the size of the squash, until the flesh is very soft when pierced with a fork.

3. Place the tofu in a medium bowl and mash it roughly with a fork.

4. Combine the onion and 2 tablespoons water in a large sauté pan. Cook over medium-high heat for 3 minutes to sweat the onion.

5. Add the tofu and 2 tablespoons more water to the pan. Cook for 8 minutes, or until the tofu begins to brown. (Use a wooden spoon or spatula to gently break up the tofu a bit more while it's cooking.) You want the tofu to really brown, so resist adding more water at this stage.

6. Add the chopped tomatoes and tomato purée. Stir gently to combine. Cook for 8 to 10 minutes, until the juices from the tomato have mostly evaporated.

7. Add the basil, oregano, nutritional yeast, and spinach, and stir to combine with the tofu mixture. Cover, reduce the heat to low, and cook for another 10 minutes, or until the spinach is just wilted but still bright green.

8. When the squash is done, flip the halves cut-side up and set aside until cool enough to handle without burning your fingers. Use a fork to scrape out the seeds, discard, then scrape out ½ cup of the squash flesh from each half and set the scraped halves aside. Add the flesh to the tofu mixture and stir to combine. (If your pan is getting full, you can mix it all together in a large bowl.)

9. Refill each squash half with the tofu mixture. Season with salt and pepper. Garnish with additional herbs, nutritional yeast, or parmesan, if desired, then serve. Store any remaining filling in an airtight container in the refrigerator for 3 to 5 days.

NOTE: If onions and tomatoes are too acidic for your stomach, you can easily leave out the onions and replace the fresh tomatoes with diced or grated zucchini.

SOURDOUGH FOR THE SOUL

Baking sourdough bread has increased in popularity in recent years, but true sourdough bread, so-called because it is made with a fermented starter more than because of its flavor, is an ancient recipe. Its nourishing properties are manifold—the preparation of the flour-and-water starter, which rises and bubbles as if by magic (aka science); the full-body experience of kneading; the patience that's cultivated from letting the dough rest and rise, then rest and rise some more; and of course, there's the incredible aroma that wafts through the house while it's baking, the unique satisfaction of slicing into a golden loaf, the tangy scent tickling your nose, and the instantly satisfying feeling in your mouth and belly with each crispy-chewy bite. (Hungry yet?)

For our friends with celiac disease, traditional sourdough bread made with wheat and/or rye flour is, alas, still off the table, but if you have a less severe sensitivity to gluten (or just suspect you do), give sourdough a try. The natural fermented base will feed your gut microbiome, making the proteins in the wheat easier to digest. Baking and breaking bread are also deeply healing rituals, whether you practive them all on your own or with loved ones around a bountiful table.

SPINACH ARTICHOKE CASHEW DIP

PREP TIME: 20 MINUTES, PLUS OVERNIGHT SOAKING   **COOK TIME:** 20 MINUTES   **SERVES** 8 TO 10

1 tablespoon extra-
virgin olive oil

⅔ cup chopped shallot
(1 medium)

1 tablespoon grated
fresh garlic

1 cup cashews,
soaked in cool water
overnight (see Note)

2 tablespoons
nutritional yeast

1 tablespoon white miso
paste

1 tablespoon tahini,
preferably homemade
(page 47)

⅓ cup apple cider
vinegar

⅛ teaspoon cayenne
pepper

½ teaspoon sea salt

½ teaspoon freshly
ground black pepper

3½ to 4 cups chopped
spinach (1 bunch)

1 (8.5-ounce) can
artichoke hearts,
drained, each heart
cut into 6 pieces

3 cups finely chopped
broccoli florets

⅓ cup Plant Parmesan
(page 50)

Socializing can be both a stressor on the nervous system. If you're someone with health or dietary concerns, then bringing a dish you know you'll love to a gathering is one way to ensure you get fed well at any event. This riff on a classic party dip will do wonders for everyone's mood—and may even introduce you to your new best friend. Enjoy it with crudité, pita bread or chips, or as a topping for grains and roasted or stir-fried veggies.

1. Preheat the oven to 375°F.

2. Heat the olive oil in a large skillet over medium heat. Add the shallot and garlic, and sauté until fragrant, about 5 minutes.

3. Transfer the mixture to a food processor and add the soaked cashews, nutritional yeast, miso, and tahini. Blend until a coarse mixture forms. Add the vinegar, then ⅓ cup water, blending between each addition to achieve a yogurt-like consistency, thick but still pourable. Add the cayenne, salt, and black pepper, adjusting the spice level to taste, and blitz to combine.

4. In the same pan you used for the shallot and garlic, lightly steam the spinach with a splash of water until just wilted, 2 to 3 minutes.

5. Place the artichokes, steamed spinach, and broccoli in an 8-inch square baking dish, and pour the cashew sauce over the vegetables. Add 2 tablespoons of the plant parmesan, then stir to combine well. Sprinkle the remaining parmesan over the top of the dip.

6. Bake for about 20 minutes, or until the dip is warmed through and lightly golden on the top. Let cool and set before serving, about 10 minutes. Store leftovers in an airtight container in the refrigerator for 3 to 4 days.

NOTE: If you're short on time, soak the nuts in boiling water for 1 hour instead of overnight.

WARM WINTER CITRUS SALAD

PREP TIME: 5 MINUTES   **COOK TIME:** 10 MINUTES   **SERVES** 2

1 shallot, chopped

1 tablespoon whole
   coriander seeds

1 teaspoon ground
   cinnamon

1 bunch asparagus,
   chopped

1 head green-leaf
   lettuce or other
   tender lettuce, cored
   and chopped

1 large grapefruit (or
   citrus of your choice)

TAHINI MISO
DRESSING
Zest and juice of 1 lime

2 tablespoons tahini,
   preferably homemade
   (page 47)

1½ teaspoons red miso
   paste

TO SERVE
Large handful of fresh
   dill, chopped

Large handful of fresh
   parsley leaves,
   chopped

Flaky sea salt and
   freshly ground black
   pepper

"Winter" and "salad" are two words that normally wouldn't go together, at least if you're talking to an herbalist. That's because the qualities of raw foods, especially cold, light, and airy greens, can exacerbate those qualities that are already in the environment in the winter months. But who said salads have to be raw? On top of gently steamed greens, which in this case are extremely nutritive, the sour citrus fruits and grounding tahini dressing stand out even more. When you enjoy this salad in the late winter and early spring months, the bitterness and astringency of the dill and parsley will give your system a good scrub to remove any accumulating congestion, too.

1. Combine the shallot and 1 tablespoon water in a large skillet. Cook over medium-high heat until the water has evaporated and the shallot begins to brown, 3 to 5 minutes.

2. Reduce the heat to low and add the coriander and cinnamon. Stir quickly to coat the pan and toast the spices, about 10 seconds.

3. Add the asparagus and ¼ cup water. Slowly raise the heat to medium-high and cook until the asparagus starts to steam and turn bright green, 5 to 7 minutes.

4. Add the lettuce to the pan, stir to combine, and cook until the lettuce is wilted but still bright in color, about 5 minutes.

5. Meanwhile, zest the grapefruit and reserve the zest in a medium bowl for the dressing. Remove the skin and pith and slice the grapefruit crosswise into thin rounds (not segments); set aside.

6. Make the dressing: Using a fork, whisk together the lime zest, lime juice, tahini, miso paste, and reserved grapefruit zest in a small bowl. Whisk in water 1 tablespoon at a time (about 2 tablespoons total, depending on your tahini) until the dressing is the consistency of runny yogurt.

7. To serve, transfer the cooked greens to a large plate. Layer the grapefruit slices on top. Drizzle with the dressing and add the dill, parsley, and a generous amount of salt and pepper. Toss gently and serve immediately. Alternatively, store the greens, grapefruit, and dressing in separate containers in the refrigerator until ready to eat.

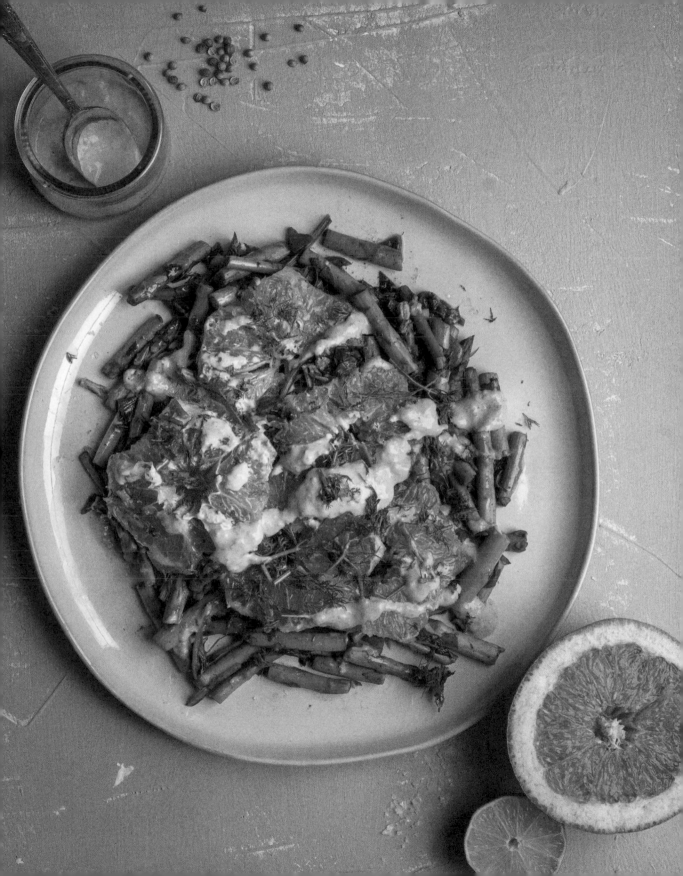

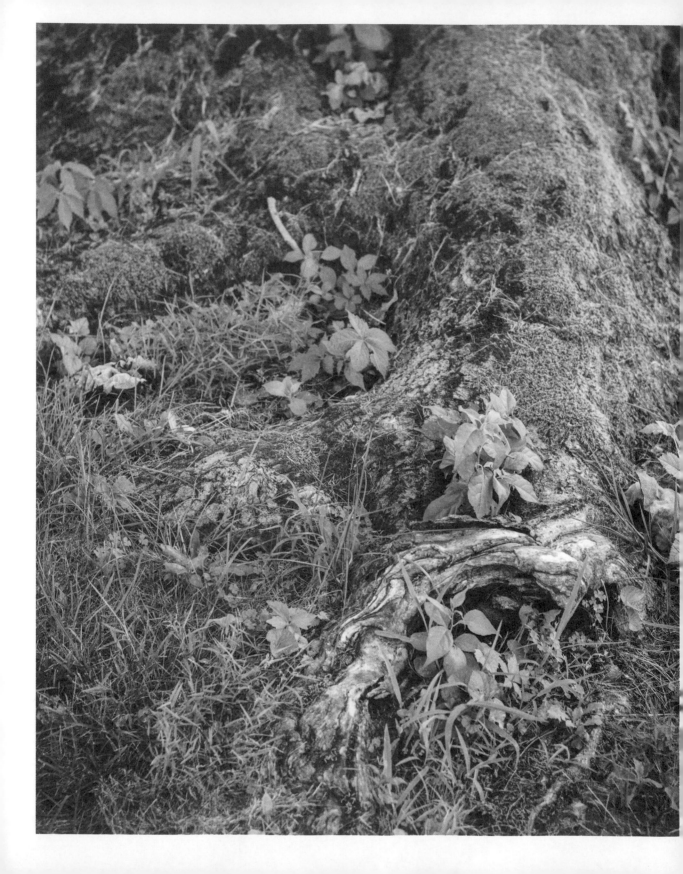

GROUNDING & CONNECTING TO PLANT ENERGY

Have you ever tried to watch a plant grow? You'd need superhuman patience to move at the pace of plants, minute by minute, but there's an important lesson to be learned about the pace of our lives from these slow-moving friends. Eating plants, and just being around them, can be a reminder to slow down and connect to their life-force, called *prana* in the yogic tradition, which is also circulating in you, too. Aligning our attention with the flow of prana is deeply nourishing for our nervous systems and can result in near instantaneous shifts in mood and mental outlook.

A wonderful way to experience prana is a simple exercise called grounding. The earth emits and transmits vibrations, and we can harness that healing energy through these basic steps:

GO OUTSIDE and find a patch of grass or soil, or anywhere you can connect directly to the earth.

REMOVE your shoes so that your feet are bare. Sink your feet into the ground. If you have the space, walk and let the natural earth massage your feet.

PAUSE—standing or sitting—and close your eyes. Connect to your surroundings with your senses. Listen to the sounds—the rustling of leaves in the wind, the song of the birds. Feel the breeze on your skin, the warmth of your breath on the space between your nose and your upper lip, the texture of the ground holding up your body. See if you can smell anything specific; perhaps the scent of grass or loamy dirt. Let your eyes soften so light comes to you, and the colors and shapes perhaps begin to blur.

HOLD this grounding space for 5 minutes in full presence of your natural surroundings. End this simple practice with 10 cleansing breaths, fully inhaling the vibrations of the earth, and exhaling any stress or worries.

WHITE BEAN CELERY ROOT SOUP WITH THYME & ROSEMARY

PREP TIME: 15 MINUTES **COOK TIME:** 50 MINUTES **SERVES** 6

- **1 tablespoon extra-virgin olive oil**
- **1 medium shallot, diced**
- **3 garlic cloves, grated**
- **1 teaspoon brown mustard seed**
- **4½ cups cubed peeled celery root**
- **2 cups cubed peeled white turnip**
- **1½ teaspoons chopped fresh thyme**
- **1½ teaspoons chopped fresh rosemary**
- **¼ teaspoon sea salt, plus more for seasoning**
- **¼ teaspoon freshly ground black pepper, plus more for seasoning**
- **1 cup dried white beans, soaked overnight**
- **4 cups vegetable broth**
- **1 bunch green Swiss chard, cut into ribbons**

The musky herbs at the heart of this soup are known for their effects on memory and cognition, as well as stress-related digestive problems. Their astringent properties are also great at scrubbing the body of unwanted toxins, mucus, and congestion, and their antimicrobial volatile oils can keep out germs. When paired with the bitter and astringent root vegetables, which have a lightening and toning effect on the body's tissues, you have a recipe to maintain current health and promote future health, which is especially important during the winter-to-spring transition.

---

1. Combine the olive oil, shallot, garlic, and mustard seed in a large pot or Dutch oven and cook over medium-low heat for 5 minutes, or until the mustard seeds are popping and fragrant.

2. Add the celery root and turnip to the pot, stir to combine, and cook for another 5 minutes.

3. Add the thyme, rosemary, salt, pepper, beans, broth, and 5 cups water to the pot. Raise the heat to high to bring to a boil, then reduce the heat to low, cover, and simmer for 35 minutes. Add the chard, cover, and simmer for another 10 minutes, or until the greens are just wilted, but still bright, and the beans are very soft. Remove from the heat, and season with additional salt and pepper to serve.

JACKFRUIT TACOS

PREP TIME: 15 MINUTES   **COOK TIME:** 15 MINUTES   **SERVES** 4

JACKFRUIT FILLING

1 lemongrass stalk

1 tablespoon Herbal
Cooking Oil (page 58)

½ yellow onion, sliced

1 (20-ounce) can green
jackfruit in water or
brine, drained and
rinsed (Trader Joe's
brand recommended)

3 garlic cloves, minced

½ cup vegetable broth
or water

1 tablespoon agave
nectar

1 teaspoon chili powder

1 teaspoon sea salt

½ teaspoon ground
cumin

½ teaspoon smoked
paprika

4 corn tortillas or hard
taco shells

1 avocado, sliced

¼ cup chopped fresh
cilantro

¼ cup loosely packed
chopped fresh lemon
balm

¼ cup loosely packed
thinly sliced red onion

¼ cup watermelon
radishes, thinly sliced

1 lime, sliced into
4 wedges

Savory Cashew Cream
(page 48)

Tacos are a beloved symbol of culinary connection and simplicity. The filling of jackfruit infused with herbal flavors gives the old favorite a new twist—one of nourishment and plant-based flavor, so you can relax and unwind in the company of food (and people) you love.

1. Make the filling: Remove the tough outer layers of the lemongrass stalk and cut off the bottom bulb. Trim and discard the tougher top portion of the stalk, leaving just the softer white bottom. Mince the lemongrass and set aside.

2. Heat the herbal cooking oil in a large skillet over medium-high heat. Stir in the onion and cook until translucent and brown, about 5 minutes.

3. Meanwhile, thinly slice the jackfruit, starting at the inner core and slicing toward the top edge.

4. Add the lemongrass, jackfruit, garlic, broth, agave, chili powder, salt, cumin, and paprika to the skillet and stir to combine. Reduce the heat to medium-low, cover, and simmer until the jackfruit is tender, 5 to 10 minutes.

5. Remove from the heat and use a potato masher to shred the jackfruit filling in the pan.

6. To serve, warm the tortillas or taco shells in a separate, dry skillet over medium heat for 1 minute on each side, or in the microwave for 30 seconds. Assemble the tacos with jackfruit filling, avocado, cilantro, lemon balm, red onion, radishes, a squeeze of lime juice, and cashew cream.

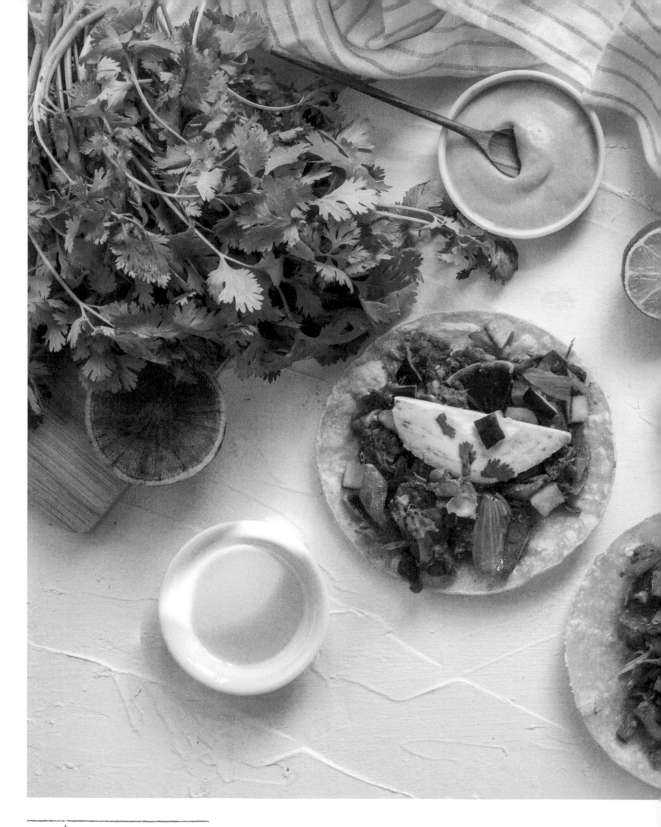

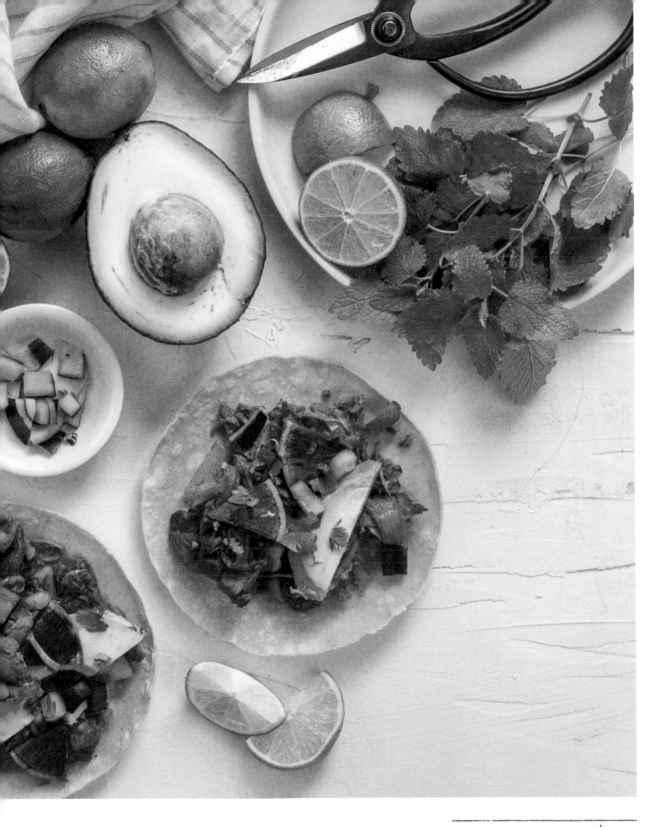

SUPER SEED SQUARES

PREP TIME: 15 MINUTES, PLUS 1 HOUR FREEZING TIME   **MAKES** 36 SQUARES

¼ cup chia seeds

⅔ cup warm water

½ cup Soaked Dates (page 48)

¼ cup coconut oil, melted

½ cup chopped raw almonds

½ cup chopped raw walnuts

½ cup raw hulled sunflower seeds

½ cup raw hulled pumpkin seeds

½ cup white hulled sesame seeds

½ cup chopped dried apricots

½ cup raw cacao nibs or chopped nondairy dark chocolate

¼ cup unsweetened coconut flakes

2 tablespoons flax meal

1½ tablespoons pure maple syrup

1½ tablespoons mucuna powder

1 tablespoon ground cardamom

1½ teaspoons ground ginger

½ teaspoon flaky sea salt

While snacking is not generally encouraged by Ayurveda (remember the Rule of Threes on page 72), ignoring hunger between meals is not a good thing, either. And when hanger strikes, our bodies, minds, and the people around us all suffer! These superfood super seed squares are the perfect antidote to energy crashes and potential stress explosions, and are even great as a quick breakfast (if you absolutely cannot sit down to eat; again, head over to page 79 for a reminder of why we don't want to eat on the go). They combine the best sources of high-quality, dense, grounding nutrition—nuts and seeds—in the perfect proportion, and a kiss of natural sweetness to help the medicine go down.

1. Combine the chia seeds with the warm water in a small bowl and let stand for 10 minutes, until set.

2. Purée the dates in a food processor or blender to make a thick paste. Transfer to a small bowl, add the coconut oil, and stir together to a uniform consistency.

3. In a separate medium bowl, stir together the almonds, walnuts, sunflower seeds, pumpkin seeds, sesame seeds, apricots, cacao nibs, coconut flakes, flax meal, and maple syrup. Add the mucuna, cardamom, ginger, and salt, and stir well. Add the chia mixture, then the date-coconut paste, stirring well after each addition.

4. Line an 8-inch square baking pan with reusable parchment. Spread the seed mixture into an even layer over the prepared pan and freeze for 1 hour. Use the parchment to lift the bars from the pan and cut into squares. Store in an airtight container in the refrigerator for up to 1 week or in the freezer for up to 2 months.

SAVORY SAGE & FLOWER TEA BISCUITS

PREP TIME: 25 MINUTES   **COOK TIME:** 30 MINUTES   **MAKES** 20 BISCUITS

1 tablespoon flax meal

½ cup almond meal

½ cup chickpea flour

½ cup oat pulp (left over from making oat mylk, page 43, or Plain Cashew Cream, page 48)

¼ cup cornmeal

½ teaspoon orange zest

3 tablespoons fresh orange juice

2 tablespoons chopped fresh sage

1½ teaspoons chopped fresh lavender leaves

⅛ teaspoon ground cloves

½ teaspoon sea salt

20 to 24 edible flowers (see Note)

The quality of a meal depends on the foods you eat, yes, but also on whom you eat with. Good company can be an essential ingredient in your diet if you're experiencing a low or inconsistent mood. So sharing these pretty—and satisfying—biscuits and a cup of tea (we recommend the Lavender, Chamomile & Rose Tea on page 157) with someone you love might just be one of the most nourishing things you could do for your mental health. Unlike traditional sweet cookies, which can exacerbate the heavying qualities of loneliness and depression, these tea biscuits showcase bright flavors and ingredients that overall lighten the body and mind through taste and sight. While the citrus and clove provide a warming, stimulating kick, the sage and lavender mellow things out with calming, woodsy notes. Whether you're savoring these biscuits in slow, mindful bites or admiring how beautiful they are on a serving plate, your whole body will thank you for indulging in these humbly nourishing treats.

1. Preheat the oven to 350°F. Line a baking sheet with reusable parchment.

2. Stir together the flax meal and 3 tablespoons hot water in a large bowl and let stand for 5 minutes, or until thickened.

3. Add the almond meal, chickpea flour, oat pulp, cornmeal, orange zest, orange juice, 1 tablespoon of the sage, the lavender, cloves, and salt to the bowl with the flax. Stir well to combine.

4. Place the dough between two pieces of reusable parchment and roll it out to ⅛-inch thickness. Use the mouth of a glass jar or measuring cup to cut out 2¼-inch rounds (it's okay if the diameter isn't precise). Place each biscuit on the prepared baking sheet, then gather the scraps of dough and repeat, until you have used all the dough. Press an edible flower into the top of each biscuit.

5. Bake for 15 minutes, or until the bottoms of the biscuits are just browned. Turn off the oven and prop open the door with the handle of a wooden spoon. Let the biscuits dry out in the oven for 15 minutes. Remove from the oven and let cool completely. Store in an airtight container in the refrigerator for up to 1 week.

NOTE: Can't find edible flowers? Use dry herbal flowers from your Kitchen Apothecary (page 23)—calendula, rose petals, lavender, and sage are all pretty options to press into these biscuits.

CHAI BROWN RICE PUDDING WITH MUCUNA

PREP TIME: 10 MINUTES   **COOK TIME:** 25 MINUTES   **SERVES** 6 TO 8

1 tablespoon dried
  oatstraw

1 Madagascar vanilla
  bean

1 cup uncooked short-
  grain brown rice,
  soaked for 30 minutes

¼ cup raisins

2 cinnamon sticks

6 whole green
  cardamom pods,
  gently crushed

1 tablespoon grated
  fresh ginger

1 teaspoon ground
  nutmeg, plus more
  for garnish

½ teaspoon freshly
  ground black pepper

1 cup light coconut milk

Ground cinnamon,
  for garnish

2 tablespoons Sweet
  Cashew Cream
  (page 48), plus
  more for garnish

Rice pudding is one of those desserts that can feel like a hug going down and a rock in your belly a few minutes after the last bite. When you find yourself craving comfort food for mood or energy imbalances that won't upset your digestion, try this herb-infused pudding. Energizing chai spices balance the sweet and grounding base of the rice, which gets creamier from baking in the oven, and is packed with more nutrition from the fiber-full brown rice and coconut milk. And in the spirit of all foods being healing any time of day, there's no reason to enjoy this only for dessert—it makes a great breakfast, brunch, or snack as well.

1. Preheat the oven to 350°F.

2. Place the oatstraw in a tea infuser, or directly in 2 cups of hot, but not boiling, water. Steep for 10 minutes, then remove the tea infuser or strain the tea through a fine-mesh sieve and discard the solids.

3. Split the vanilla bean in half lengthwise and scrape out the seeds and pulp.

4. Combine the tea, vanilla bean seeds and pod, rice, raisins, cinnamon, cardamom, ginger, nutmeg, pepper, and coconut milk in a large ovenproof pot or Dutch oven. Bring to a boil over medium heat, then cook for 5 minutes.

5. Remove the pot from the heat, cover, and transfer to the oven. Bake for 20 minutes, or until the rice is very thick and creamy. Stir in the cashew cream. Let cool slightly; discard the vanilla bean and cinnamon sticks before serving.

6. Divide into bowls, and top with additional cinnamon, nutmeg, or cashew cream, as desired, and serve.

OATS (AVENA SATIVA)

NOURISHING HERBS

You're probably familiar with oats as a cereal grain—rolled, quick, steel-cut, etc. But did you know there are other ways to cultivate, use, and consume oats? Milky oats, oatstraw, and the mature oat grain are all different parts of the oat plant, *Avena sativa L*. Milky oats are a nutritive substance exuded by the immature florets, or the top part of the plant. Oatstraw is the grassy stalk and offers more long-term tonic support than milky oats. In any form, oats are a potent nervine and can "feed" a run-down nervous system.

ALTERNATE NOSTRIL BREATHING

(NADI SHODHANA PRANAYAMA)

*P*ranayama means directing the life-force energy (known as *prana*) primarily by bringing attention to our breath. In this exercise, we are balancing the two dominant energies in the body: masculine/sun/*yang* and feminine/moon/*yin*. All of us, regardless of gender, have both energies, but when one gets out of balance, we can experience symptoms such as anxiety, depression, or mood swings. This practice takes just 5 to 10 minutes and can help bring the mind to a place of ease and contentment, which we call *sattva* in Ayurveda (see page 154 for more on sattva).

Come to a comfortable seated position, cross-legged on the floor or on a chair. If you are on the floor, you may wish to support yourself on a blanket, pillow, or cushion. You may keep your eyes open or close them, as you prefer. Let your left hand rest on your left leg, palm facing up. Bring your right index finger and middle finger into the palm of your hand, so the thumb and ring finger are free. Lift your right arm so the elbow is out to the side and bring your right thumb to your right nostril and your right ring finger to your left nostril.

Apply gentle pressure with your thumb to close off your right nostril, then breathe in through your free left nostril. Switch, closing your left nostril and breathing out through your right nostril. Breathe in through your right nostril, then switch again, closing your right nostril and breathing out through your left. That is one round.

Continue alternating the breath, slowly and gently, for 5 to 10 minutes, ending with breathing out through your left nostril. Relax your right hand on your leg and take a full cycle of breath through both nostrils. Slowly open your eyes, if they were closed, and notice how you feel. Practice *nadi shodhana pranayama* (alternate nostril breathing) as part of your morning meditation, before bed, or whenever you feel you need a moment of clarity.

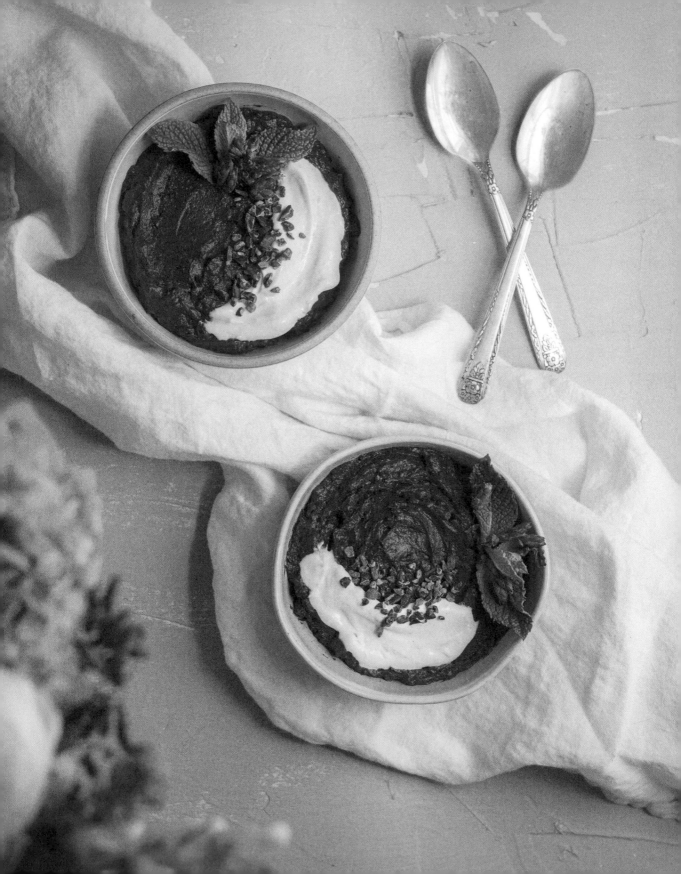

MINT CACAO AVOCADO PUDDING

PREP TIME: 10 MINUTES   **SERVES** 6 TO 8

2 cups avocado flesh (from 2 medium avocados)

1¼ cups Soaked Dates (page 48)

⅓ cup raw cacao powder

1½ tablespoons unsweetened coconut flakes

2 tablespoons chopped fresh mint leaves, plus more for garnish (see Note)

Whipped Coconut Cream with Marshmallow Root (page 49) or Cashew Cream (page 48), for garnish

Flaky sea salt, for garnish

Spoons are highly undervalued in our eating culture, especially when you think about how much power and goodness can come from a spoonful (or five) of this pudding. Unlike the boxed pudding mix some of us grew up with, this recipe harnesses the power of whole-food ingredients to create a creamy, sweet, grounding yet uplifting treat that's quick enough to make when a craving strikes or a last-minute party invitation comes along and you need a dessert to bring. If you're looking for an instant chocolate fix, you can easily reduce the recipe to make a single serving (though why wouldn't you want extra?). You can also adjust the quantity of mint depending on your tolerance of this potent herb—start with less if your stomach is sensitive to it, since you can always add more later.

1. Combine the avocado and dates in a food processor. Blitz until smooth, about 2 minutes.

2. Add the cacao, coconut flakes, and mint leaves. Blitz until well combined, stopping to scrape down the sides to incorporate all the cacao, another 2 to 3 minutes. Taste to adjust the mint.

3. Spoon the pudding into bowls. Top with a dollop of coconut cream or cashew cream, a sprinkle of flaky sea salt, and additional mint, as desired.

NOTE: There will be a few small flecks of mint in the final dish. If you prefer a completely smooth pudding, omit the mint that gets blended into the pudding and use ½ teaspoon pure mint extract to flavor it instead.

ADAPTOGENIC DOUBLE CHOCOLATE BROWNIES

PREP TIME: 10 MINUTES, PLUS 30 MINUTES COOLING TIME   **COOK TIME:** 35 MINUTES
MAKES 9 LARGE BROWNIES OR 16 SMALL BROWNIES

¼ cup flax meal

½ cup warm water

1½ cups coconut sugar

½ cup non-expeller-pressed palm shortening, melted

1 tablespoon pure vanilla extract, preferably homemade (page 44)

1 cup gluten-free measure-for-measure flour blend (King Arthur brand preferred)

2 tablespoons apoptogenic mushroom powder

Scant 1 cup raw cacao powder

2 teaspoons raw cacao nibs

1 teaspoon baking powder

½ teaspoon sea salt

1 cup dark nondairy chocolate chips or dark chocolate chunks

When in doubt, bring brownies. Whether you're heading to a celebration with loved ones, or just want to celebrate yourself, these delicious brownies have everything you need to feel at ease and nourished, thanks to a healthy dose of adaptogens. Cacao nibs mixed into the batter gives the brownies a nutrient boost, whereas the dark chocolate chunks on top deliver on eye appeal and sweetness. Warming, tonifying, and detoxifying, the herbs used in these ultra-fudgy brownies promote longevity, so the effects of these treats last long after you lick the last crumble out of the pan.

1. Preheat the oven to 350°F. Line an 8-inch square pan with reusable parchment, letting the parchment overhang two sides by 2 to 3 inches (so it's easy to lift out the brownies when they're done).

2. Stir together the flax meal and the warm water in a small bowl and let stand for 5 minutes, or until thickened.

3. Add the coconut sugar to the bowl with the flax and whisk to combine with the melted shortening. Stir in the vanilla.

4. Add the mushroom powder to a 1-cup measuring cup, then fill the rest of the cup with cacao powder. Add to the bowl with the flour blend, then add the cacao nibs, baking powder, and salt. Stir until just combined. The batter should be very thick. Fold in ½ cup of the chocolate chips or chunks.

5. Pour the batter into the prepared pan and evenly smooth it out to the corners using a spatula or your hands. Sprinkle the remaining ½ cup chocolate chips or chunks over the batter. Bake for 30 to 35 minutes—they will still look a little underbaked and fudgy when they come out of the oven. Let cool in the pan for 15 minutes.

6. Using the overhanging parchment, carefully lift the brownies from the pan and set them on a flat surface to cool for another 15 minutes, or until they firm up. (This double cooling helps the brownies achieve the right texture.) Slice into squares and serve with your favorite glass of plant mylk.

REISHI *(GANODERMA LUCIDUM)*

Adaptogenic mushrooms are becoming more and more popular these days, but reishi has been a favorite of herbalists for centuries. Easily grown in the U.S., reishi has a combined sweet-bitter flavor profile that relieves anxiety by lifting the spirits (sweet) and calming the mind (bitter). It's best taken in the evening to support restful sleep, but also has strong short- and long-term effects on the immune system, mental clarity, and is anti-inflammatory. While reishi is popularly known as the "king of mushrooms," we think of it more as a queen.

HAPPY LEMON BARS

PREP TIME: 20 MINUTES, PLUS 2 TO 3 DAYS INFUSION TIME AND 2 HOURS CHILLING
COOK TIME: 40 MINUTES   **MAKES** 9 LARGE BARS OR 16 SMALL BARS

CHAMOMILE SYRUP (SEE NOTE)
1 tablespoon dried chamomile flowers

1 cup pure maple syrup

OAT CRUST
1 cup gluten-free rolled oats

1 cup raw slivered almonds

⅓ cup coconut sugar

¼ teaspoon sea salt

¼ cup coconut oil, melted

LEMON FILLING
3 tablespoons aquafaba (see Note)

1 teaspoon pure vanilla extract, preferably homemade (page 44)

1 tablespoon lemon zest

Juice of 1 large lemon

1 cup coconut cream (preferably Nature's Charm; see Note page 49)

1½ teaspoons cornstarch

¼ teaspoon sea salt

Confectioners' sugar, for dusting (optional)

Lemons are the first fruit that come to mind when we think of a "happy" food. In a classic sweet treat like lemon bars, their vibrant color, uplifting smell, and enlivening taste combine to make for a pan of happiness you'll be as eager to share as to enjoy yourself.

***

1. Make the chamomile syrup: Combine the chamomile and maple syrup in a jar, seal the lid, and allow the herbal properties to infuse for 2 to 3 days in the refrigerator. Strain with a fine-mesh strainer to remove the chamomile and store the jar in the refrigerator for up to 1 month. (You will have more syrup than you need for the recipe.)

2. Preheat the oven to 350°F. Line an 8-inch square baking dish with reusable parchment, letting the parchment overhang two sides by 2 to 3 inches (so it's easy to lift out the lemon bars when they're done).

3. Make the oat crust: Combine the oats, almonds, coconut sugar, and salt in a food processor and blitz until it breaks down into a coarse meal. Transfer to a medium bowl and stir in 1 tablespoon of the chamomile syrup and the melted coconut oil until evenly combined. Press the crust mixture into the prepared baking dish, covering the bottom evenly and pressing the crust into the corners. Bake for 15 to 20 minutes, until golden.

4. Meanwhile, make the filling: Whisk together the aquafaba, 2 tablespoons of the chamomile syrup, the vanilla, lemon zest, and lemon juice in a medium bowl. Whisk in the coconut cream, then mix for about 5 minutes, until smooth. Slowly add the cornstarch and salt and whisk until there are no lumps.

5. Remove the crust from the oven and pour the filling evenly over the top. Return the baking dish to the oven and bake for 15 to 20 minutes, until the center jiggles but the edges are firm. Remove from the oven and let the lemon bars cool to room temperature. (This helps prevent cracking and separating.) Refrigerate the cooled lemon bars for at least 2 hours.

6. Dust the pan with confectioners' sugar if desired, cut into squares, and serve.

NOTE: For an extra dose of calm, use the leftover chamomile maple syrup on Vanilla Sweet Potato Banana Pancakes (page 116), or in any dish for which you use maple syrup as a sweetener.
   Aquafaba is the liquid that's produced from cooking chickpeas. Slightly viscous, it has the consistency of egg whites and is often used to add fluff to vegan baking. You can make your own from our Dried Beans recipe (page 51), or simply strain from a can of chickpeas.

PASSIONFLOWER MOCKTAIL

PREP TIME: 15 MINUTES   **SERVES** 2

2 tablespoons dried tulsi

2 tablespoons dried passionflower

½ cup fresh tart cherries, pitted, plus more for garnish

1 teaspoon pure vanilla extract, preferably homemade (page 44)

3 drops of Herbal Vinegar Bitters (page 59)

1 tablespoon raw honey

1 cup ice

Sea salt, to rim the glasses (optional)

Need to relax and unwind after a long day? Passionflower's powerful sedative properties combined with tulsi's adaptogenic qualities will help the body resist stressors and relieve any tension that may be lingering. The tart cherries and vinegar bitters add some punchy flavor to lighten the mood, making this a fun party beverage. Serve your guests a glass of peace and tranquility with this lovely drink.

1. Bring 3 cups water to a boil in a small saucepan over high heat. Add the tulsi and passionflower, reduce the heat to medium-low, cover, and simmer for 10 minutes. Let cool.

2. Meanwhile, combine the cherries and vanilla in a blender and purée until smooth. Transfer the purée to a jar or shaker and set aside.

3. Strain the tea through a fine-mesh sieve into the jar or shaker with the cherry purée. Add the vinegar bitters, honey, and ice. Cover and shake well.

4. Fill a shallow bowl with 2 tablespoons water and spread the salt over a small plate or small shallow bowl. Dip the rim of 2 glasses in the water, then into the salt, turning it to coat. Add ice to each glass and pour the mocktail into the glasses. Garnish with additional cherries, if desired, and serve.

NOURISHING HERBS

PASSIONFLOWER *(PASSIFLORA INCARNATA)*

Passionflower, a perennial climbing vine with striking flowers, is a nervine relaxant and strong herbal sedative. Its use dates back thousands of years to prehistoric times, and it is cherished for its ability to nourish friendships and peace. The leaves, stems, and flowers are traditionally used as a tea or in a tincture, as we use it here. Passionflower is a great addition to a mocktail because of its relaxing properties, something people often turn to alcohol for—those properties are strong in this special plant, so enjoy in moderation.

LEMON BALM LEMONADE

PREP TIME: 5 MINUTES   **SERVES** 8

8 lemons, halved

½ cup fresh lemon balm, chopped

1 to 2 cups agave nectar, to taste (see Note)

Lemon balm is best known for its nervine relaxant properties, meaning it provides a supportive feeling of calm and well-being. Enjoy it in a cool glass of this lemonade as a balm to the mind and soul.

1. Use a citrus press to juice the lemons into a 2-quart jug or jar. Set aside the juiced lemon halves.

2. Add the lemon balm and agave to the lemon juice and stir.

3. Add 8 cups water and the reserved lemon halves. Mix well.

4. Pour into glasses over ice and enjoy chilled.

NOTE: Adjust the amount of agave nectar based on the sweetness level preferred—1 cup will be very mildly sweetened, whereas 2 cups will make a more traditionally sweet lemonade.

	LEMON BALM (MELISSA OFFICINALIS)
NOURISHING HERBS	Delicate and fragrant, lemon balm adds a hint of uplifting citrus scent to food, drinks, and even cosmetics. It offers mild sedative and digestive support, with the overall effect of relaxing the nervous system. We think you'll love this herb, and not only for its heart-shaped leaves; its genus name, *Melissa*, is the Greek word for "honeybee," so called after the bees' affection for its heavenly aroma.

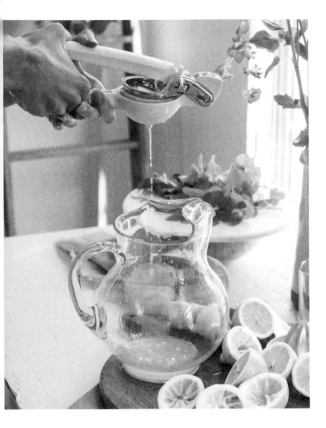
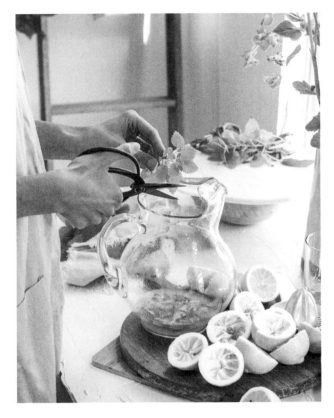
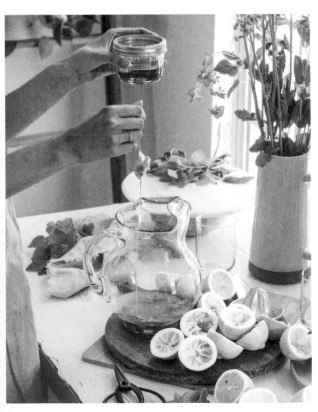
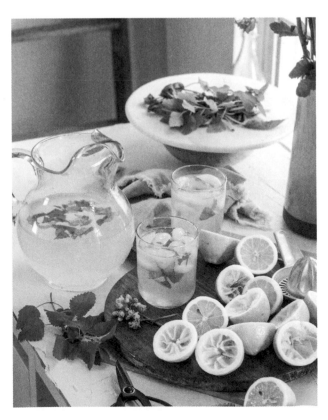

CREAMY CHAI LATTE

COOK TIME: 10 MINUTES   **MAKES** 1 GENEROUS MUG

1 heaping tablespoon chopped fresh ginger

2 cinnamon sticks

6 whole green cardamom pods, lightly crushed

4 whole cloves

2 star anise pods

1 tablespoon dried oatstraw

½ teaspoon ground nutmeg

¼ teaspoon freshly ground black pepper

½ cup oat mylk or coconut mylk, preferably homemade (page 43)

½ teaspoon raw honey

Chai, how do we love thee? Although "chai" means "tea" of any kind, chai in the way most Westerners think of it—that spicy-sweet goodness that signals the start of fall—has its own litany of benefits. While the spice combination stimulates and heals the digestive system, which houses our immunity and emotions in addition to breaking down food, the lingering aroma and warming aftereffect on the body means that just one cup will leave an impression on your nervous system. Steeping the whole herbs and spices off the heat, rather than boiling them in the water, also helps to release their volatile oils, which is where all their healing potential lies.

1. Combine the ginger, cinnamon, cardamom, cloves, star anise, oatstraw, nutmeg, pepper, and 2 cups water in a medium saucepan. Bring to a boil over high heat, then remove from the heat, cover, and let steep for 8 minutes.

2. Add the mylk and return to a low heat until the mylk is gently frothing along the sides of the pan, 2 to 3 minutes.

3. Strain the tea into a large mug, let cool slightly, and stir in the honey.

CAYENNE CACAO WITH TAHINI

COOK TIME: 10 MINUTES   **MAKES** 1 GENEROUS MUG

2½ tablespoons raw cacao powder

½ teaspoon ashwagandha root powder

½ teaspoon mucuna powder

⅛ teaspoon cayenne pepper

1 cinnamon stick

½ cup oat mylk, preferably homemade (page 43)

1½ teaspoons tahini, preferably homemade (page 47)

1½ teaspoons pure maple syrup

If you don't associate chocolate with pleasure, by all means feel free to move on to the next recipe. But we're banking on the idea that you're like us, and as soon as stress comes knocking, there's only one thing that will answer the door: cacao. Naturally stimulating and arousing to the nervous system and beyond, cacao is a great way to satisfy the unsatisfiables in your world. But add in adaptogenic ashwagandha and mucuna, pungent cayenne and cinnamon, and creamy oats and tahini, and you've got yourself a cup full of multifaceted healing nourishment. This cacao has a real kick, so if you're not used to spices, go easy on the cayenne—start with barely a pinch, then adjust up to ⅛ teaspoon.

1. Whisk together the cacao powder and 1 cup water in a small saucepan to make a smooth paste.

2. Add the ashwagandha, mucuna, cayenne, and cinnamon. Bring to a boil over medium heat, then reduce the heat to low and simmer for 5 minutes. Add the mylk and simmer for another 2 minutes or until the mylk is gently frothing along the sides of the pan.

3. Remove from the heat and stir. Pour the cacao into a mug. Blitz with a handheld frother or whisk vigorously with a fork or electric frother. Stir in the tahini and maple syrup.

AYURVEDIC PSYCHOLOGY

SATTVA, RAJAS & TAMAS

Ayurveda describes the mind as having three possible states: *sattva* (balanced, harmonious, clear), *rajas* (active, restless, aggressive), and *tamas* (inert, dark, decaying). Food is one of many things that contribute to our state of mind, so we can look to the qualities of food, in addition to factors in our environment, as a possible root cause for mental imbalance. Sour, salty, or spicy foods tend to increase rajas, which can be healing when you're experiencing lower energy or mood as a way to elevate us out of tamas and move toward sattva. However, if you're already feeling anxious or high-strung, you might choose foods with more tamasic qualities, to bring a sense of grounding and density to the system; these include bitter, astringent, and sweet tastes (natural sweeteners, like honey and maple syrup, as well as stewed fruits and root vegetables), and foods like oils, nuts and seeds, grains, and mushrooms. Sattvic foods will promote balance and integration throughout the system, and as you might expect have the qualities we look for in a balanced and integrated lifestyle—foods that are organic, locally grown and seasonal, mostly plant-based, and cooked with love.

In the same way that we will encounter all the tastes—in food and in life—we need to have sattva, rajas, and tamas in our minds, and their levels are constantly changing throughout the day and year (think: rajas gets you up in the morning, tamas puts you to sleep, and sattva helps you make decisions in line with your values). If you're noticing that you are tending toward one quality of mind more often than not, notice if there are similar patterns in your food and start to incorporate more of the opposite. Playing with how you spice and season basic ingredients—like rice, vegetables, or even cacao—can completely alter how they taste to your mind and your mouth, increasing the level of nourishment and joy you derive from your food, and expanding what it means to use food as medicine.

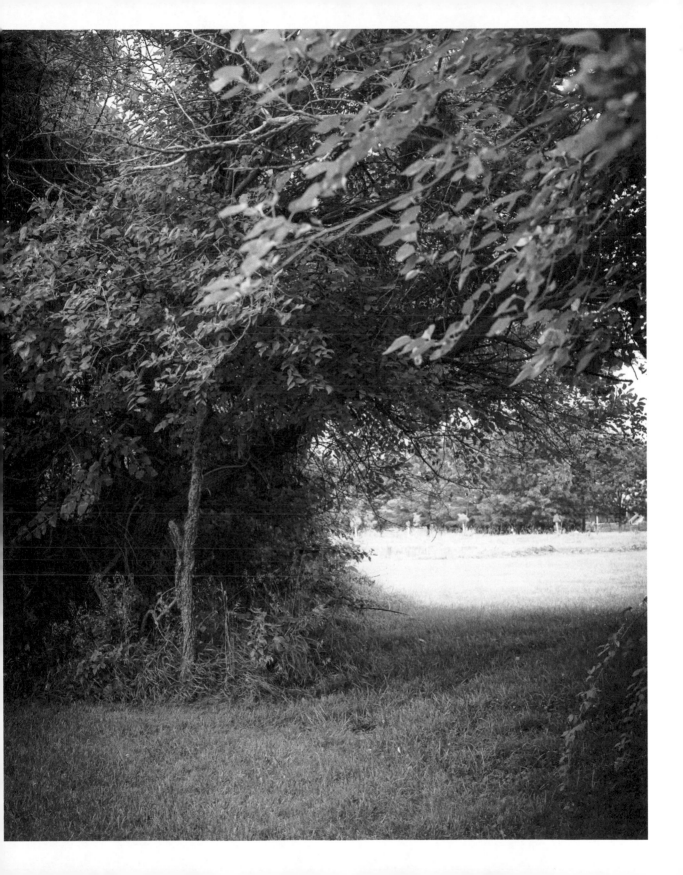

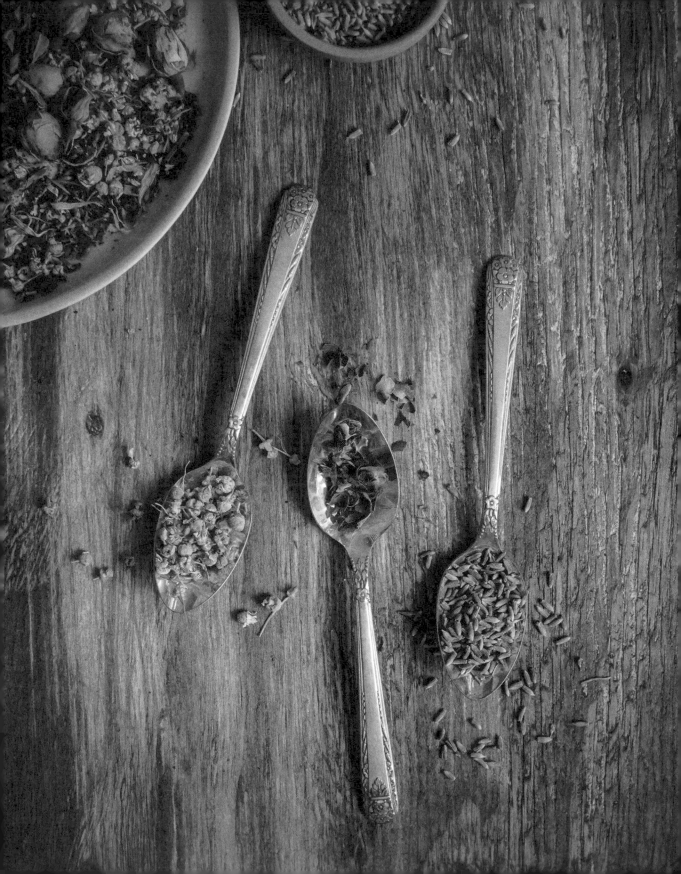

LAVENDER, CHAMOMILE & ROSE TEA

PREP TIME: 15 MINUTES **SERVES** 1

½ teaspoon dried culinary-grade lavender

½ teaspoon dried chamomile flowers

½ teaspoon dried culinary-grade rose petals

1 teaspoon raw honey or other sweetener, or to taste

Think of this tea as a warm herbal hug. Lavender, chamomile, and roses are gentle nervine relaxants, which means preparing and sipping them in tea form provides emotional support as an act of loving self-care. You can strain the herbs before you drink the tea, but it's also fun to leave them in and do a little tea-leaf reading at the end of your teatime ritual.

1. Bring 2 cups water to a boil in a tea kettle or small saucepan over high heat.

2. Place the lavender, chamomile, and rose petals in a tea infuser and put the infuser in a mug. Gently pour the boiling water over the herbs. Let steep for 10 minutes.

3. Remove the tea infuser or tea bag, if you like. Stir in the honey.

LAVENDER (*LAVANDULA ANGUSTIFOLIA*)

NOURISHING HERBS

Beloved for its fragrance by the early Egyptians, Greeks, and Romans, lavender was considered a superior herb for bathing, perfume, cooking, and medicine, and even named it as such—its etymological root is the Latin word *lavare*, which means "to wash." English lavender (*Lavandula angustifolia*), also known as French or Common Lavender, is the most popular form of the herb used today. Although the pleasant aroma of its gray-purple flowers make it a staple of aromatherapy, when used medicinally, lavender is carminative, sedative, bitter, and antimicrobial. This makes it an excellent support for digestion and mental health, and for cleansing of body, mind, and spirit

English folklore tells that a blend of lavender, mugwort, chamomile, and rose petals (more or less the ingredients in this tea recipe!) will attract sprites, fairies, brownies (helpful household spirits, who enjoy brownies as dessert, too), and elves—so watch out for magical encounters.

GENTLE YOGA FOR RELAXATION

At the end (or the start!) of a long day, pamper your nervous system with these gentle supported yoga postures that will circulate your energy without excess stimulation. Practice for a few minutes before bed, or any time you need a moment of calm and clarity. For extra herbal relaxation, use a lavender-scented eye pillow while you rest in the postures, or use lavender, frankincense, and/or vetiver essential oils in a diffuser while you practice.

WIND-RELIEVING POSE (*APANASANA*)   Lie down on your back on a soft surface. Draw one knee in to your chest, holding on to your shin or the back of your thigh. Take 3 to 5 rounds of breath in stillness, then 3 to 5 breaths making circles with your knee and hip. Switch legs. Then hold both knees in to your chest and make circles with your knees, keeping your awareness on the back of your pelvis (sacrum) on the ground.

SUPPORTED FISH POSE (*MATSYASANA*)   Set up two large bed pillows or a yoga bolster vertically along the center of your yoga mat or other surface. Place a folded blanket or towel at the back edge of the props for your head. Sit down right in front of the props, then gently recline backward over the props, adjusting the height of the back blanket so your neck is not stretching. Position your legs long on the ground, feet on the floor, with knees bent, or feet together and knees apart. Let your arms open to your sides or rest your hands on your body. Stay here for 5 to 10 minutes.

SUPPORTED CHILD'S POSE (*BALASANA*)   Set up a stack of pillows or two yoga blocks at the front of your space. Take a blanket or towel and fold it into a long rectangle. Make a small roll from the long side. Sit on your shins with your knees a little wider than your hips and your feet touching, releasing your seat to your heels. Take the rolled blanket and place it in the crease of your hips, pulling it snug around the outside of your legs. Lengthen your torso, then fold over your legs and the blanket. Release your forehead to the props and rest your arms in front of them in a cactus shape, palms down. Stay here for 5 to 10 minutes, breathing into the length and width of your back body.

CORPSE POSE (*SAVASANA*)   Place a blanket over your entire yoga mat. Take another blanket or towel and make a short roll or use a yoga bolster. Place your legs over the blanket roll or bolster so your knees are supported, then lie down on your mat. Let your feet roll out to the sides and rest your arms a few inches away from your body. Cover yourself with a blanket or wear a sweater or socks if you feel chilly. Scan your body from your head to your feet and taking notice of any areas of tension or holding. Visualize more breath going to those areas, like water softening the jagged edges of a rock. Stay here for 5 to 10 minutes.

HERBAL LULLABY TEA

PREP TIME: 15 MINUTES   **SERVES** 2

½ teaspoon dried
skullcap

½ teaspoon dried tulsi

½ teaspoon dried
passionflower

½ teaspoon dried
licorice root

Raw honey or other
sweetener to taste

Harness the strength of these powerful sedative herbs when the body is in fight, flight, or freeze mode and feelings of anxiety or overwhelm persist. They collectively come together to provide a sense of serenity and ease.

1. Bring 2 cups water to a boil in a tea kettle or small saucepan over high heat.

2. Place the skullcap, tulsi, passionflower, and licorice root in a tea infuser and put the infuser in a mug. Gently pour the boiling water over the herbs. Let steep for 10 minutes.

3. Remove the tea infuser. Stir in the honey.

	SKULLCAP *(SCUTELLARIA LATERIFLORA)*
NOURISHING HERBS	Herbalism doesn't always have an instant fix for health concerns, but skullcap is a noted exception. Known for its ability to bring comfort and calm to the mind during acute distress, this flowering plant has leaves that look like a soldier's helmet (hence its name)—so you might think of it as your own internal defense system. Skullcap is used most often as a nervous system tonic to support frayed nerves, a muscle relaxant, and as a sleep aid. While both American skullcap (the type used here) and Chinese skullcap are members of the mint family, Chinese skullcap (*Scutellaria baicalensis*) is a different plant, which is more bitter and is used to support the liver and the immune system.

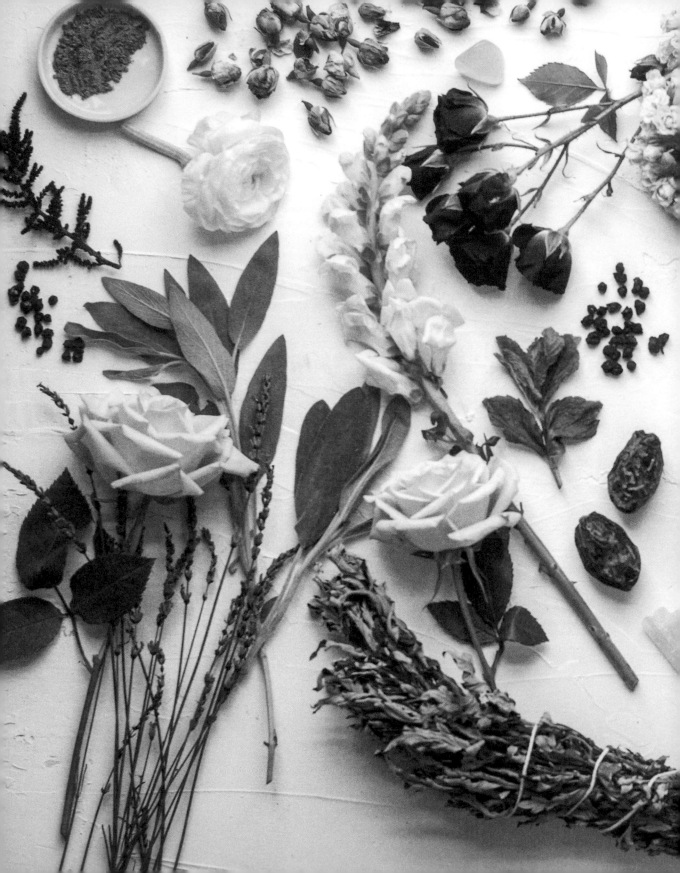

PART III

FEMALE REPRODUCTIVE HORMONAL HEALTH

Now I am a woman longing to be a
    tree, planted in a moist, dark earth
Between sunrise and sunset—

—JOY HARJO, "SPEAKING TREE"

When you think about herbs, what first comes to mind is probably something like a leaf, maybe a flower or stem. These delicate plant parts have much nutritional value, but they're only part of the story. The real action can be found a little deeper, in the seeds of the plant. All life sprouts from some form of seed, and without them there'd be none of those gorgeous leaves and flowers for us to use in our healing practices. Concentrated containers for the entire plant's journey and unique properties, seeds are tiny miracles of creation, growth, and evolution.

It's no wonder that seeds are an integral part of our herbal remedies for female reproductive hormonal balance. Like plants, women are born with a lifetime's worth of seeds (eggs, or ova) that, biologically speaking, get "planted" in the form of pregnancy. Our menstrual cycle, and what leads up to it and comes after it, are all part of our seeds' journey. But that's not the only way our lives depend on seeds. There are also the metaphorical seeds that we plant as we grow into ourselves over the course of our lives. Our activities, education, relationships, careers, homes, and spirituality are all reflections of

how our seeds' well-being—the nature of the blueprints they contain as well as how we're caring for them.

We can't talk about our reproductive systems without talking about hormones. Deeply complex and poorly understood, even by Western medicine, hormones are not explicitly discussed in Eastern medicinal texts except as parts of the many levels of metabolism (*agni* in Ayurveda) that keep things going throughout the whole body. Modern medicine often approaches conditions stemming from hormones with an isolationist mind-set—that hormones like estrogen, progesterone, and testosterone; adrenaline and cortisol; insulin; thyroid and pituitary hormones, etc., are mere chemicals that can be replaced or turned off or enhanced with a pill. But the intricate dance of these whole-system communicators isn't one that can be broken down so easily. Like we've seen throughout this book, hormones, which control everything from our sleep to our hunger to our threat and stress responses, are connected to everything else we do. And if hormones are yet another form of fire in our bodies, we know exactly how to manage them: feed them.

Both Western herbalism and Ayurveda have a number of targeted reproductive-hormone therapies that, together with diet, can support individual needs. It's beyond the scope of this book to advise specific protocols for all hormonal imbalances, so we will keep things simple and split hormones into two categories: the stimulating, heating, fight-or-flight, yang hormones of the sympathetic nervous system, and the grounding, cooling, rest-and-digest, yin hormones of the parasympathetic nervous system. When the levels of one go up, the levels of the other go down. As we discussed in Part II, our stress response—the ability to react and move quickly out of danger, and/or our ability to freeze up and protect ourselves when danger comes—rises when we have a lot of sympathetic hormones; we feel alive and "on." The body can actually convert some of its parasympathetic hormones—the ones responsible for building and nurturing, resting and digesting—in order to keep up its stress levels. This is one reason why when we experience stress for too long, especially without real danger around, we can become depleted and burned out. We simply don't have enough parasympathetic juice to maintain our state of normal functioning, or homeostasis, which includes growth, cell repair, immunity, digestion and elimination, sleep, and—you guessed it—reproduction.

When we do things to support digestion and mental health, we'll naturally affect reproduction, too, which is a great thing if you've been following along in this book with the foods and practices to build back up your yin functions. In this section, you'll find a number of ways to more specifically nourish your reproductive hormones with plants, some of which you may have heard of already (phytoestrogens, adaptogens, aphrodisiacs). The recipes here, however, are more geared toward the sentiment of rest and slowing down that will bring balance to your whole body's hormonal network, so there is more parasympathetic juice. What does that mean? Less stress. Less busyness. Less multitasking. Less restricting. Less fear. Less.

The word "less" is often used today in the context of reducing ourselves: in our physical forms, our voices, or our needs and desires. But here, we invite you to see "less" as a pathway to more. More space in the day to prepare and eat your meals, more time to spend with loved ones, rest, sleep (remember they're different), and dream of what you'll create from the seeds ripening within you. The foods here offer enjoyment, pleasure, and indulgence—which doesn't just mean sweets. They reflect beauty, ease, and harmony in how they look, smell, and taste, so those qualities can take root inside of you. It's a shift in mind-set that anyone of any gender or sexual identity can take on to welcome more creative flow into their day and life.

These recipes also support general female reproductive hormonal health, rather than for specific concerns around fertility, pregnancy, and menopause. Most herbal protocols are contraindicated during pregnancy and, as mentioned above, each woman will have her own unique history determining the way her hormones affect her fertility and menopausal experiences that are beyond the scope of this book. Please consult your healthcare provider or holistic practitioner for more personalized guidance with those goals.

The herbs in this section (see the full list starting below) fall into many overlapping categories, which you can read more about in the Herbal Actions section on page 26.

+ Adaptogenic
+ Alterative
+ Antioxidant
+ Antispasmodic
+ Aphrodisiac
+ Astringent
+ Emmenagogue
+ Phytoestrogenic
+ Tonic (adrenal and uterine)

In addition to these herbs, we love the following foods to support reproductive health with their heavying, building, and down-regulating energies and nutrients:

+ **Cacao:** an ancient superfood chock full of essential minerals (such as magnesium and iron), antioxidants, and chemical compounds that stimulate the nervous system and stabilize hormones. We recommend incorporating raw cacao regularly into your diet, or dark nondairy chocolate (over 70 percent cacao).
+ **Coconut:** all forms, including mylk, flakes, oil, butter, and water
+ **Dates**
+ **Oils:** olive, coconut, sesame, avocado
+ **Seeds:** especially pumpkin, flax, sesame, and sunflower seeds, which contain phytoestrogens and energetic properties to balance hormones (see pages 170–175 for more on seeds and your menstrual cycle). When you buy them, choose whole, raw, hulled versions from the bulk section if possible, and then you can toast or grind them yourself if needed. Store seeds in a jar or airtight container in the refrigerator or freezer up to 1 year.

ASHWAGANDHA (*WITHANIA SOMNIFERA*)	adaptogenic, adrenal tonic, aphrodisiac, astringent
ASIAN GINSENG (*PANAX GINSENG*)	adaptogenic, adrenal tonic, aphrodisiac
BLACK PEPPER (*PIPER NIGRUM*)	antioxidant
CALENDULA (*CALENDULA OFFICINALIS*)	alterative, antispasmodic, emmenagogue, phytoestrogenic (mild)
CILANTRO (*CORIANDRUM SATIVUM*)	alterative, emmenagogue
CINNAMON (*CINNAMOMUM ZEYLANICUM*)	antioxidant, astringent
CUMIN (*CUMINUM CYMINUM*)	antispasmodic, emmenagogue
ELDERBERRY (*SAMBUCUS NIGRA* SUBSP. *CANADENSIS*)	alterative, antioxidant, antispasmodic
FENNEL (*FOENICULUM VULGARE*)	phytoestrogenic
FENUGREEK (*TRIGONELLA FOENUMGRAECEUM*)	aphrodisiac, emmenagogue, uterine tonic
GINGER (*ZINGIBER OFFICINALE*)	aphrodisiac
HIBISCUS (*HIBISCUS SABDARIFFA*)	aphrodisiac, astringent, emmenagogue

FLAXSEED (*LINUM USITATISSIMUM*)	phytoestrogenic
LAVENDER (*LAVANDULA ANGUSTIFOLIA*)	antispasmodic, emmenagogue
LEMONGRASS (*CYMBOPOGON CITRATUS*)	astringent, emmenagogue
LICORICE ROOT (*GLYCYRRHIZA GLABRA*)	adaptogenic, adrenal tonic, antispasmodic, phytoestrogenic
MACA (*LEPIDIUM MEYENII*)	adaptogenic, aphrodisiac, emmenagogue, phytoestrogen
MUCUNA (*MUCUNA PRURIENS*)	adaptogenic, aphrodisiac
NETTLE (*URTICA DIOICA*)	emmenagogue, uterine tonic
NUTMEG (*MYRISTICA FRAGRANS*)	antispasmodic
OATSTRAW (*AVENA SATIVA L.*)	antioxidant, antispasmodic, aphrodisiac
PEPPERMINT (*MENTHA PIPERITA*)	antispasmodic, emmenagogue
PUMPKIN SEEDS (*CUCURBITA PEPO*)	phytoestrogenic
RED RASPBERRY LEAF (*RUBUS IDAEUS*)	astringent, emmenagogue, uterine tonic
REISHI (*GANODERMA LUCIDUM*)	adaptogenic, antioxidant
ROSE (*ROSA DAMASCENA*)	antispasmodic, aphrodisiac, emmenagogue, uterine tonic
SAGE (*SALVIA OFFICINALIS*)	astringent, emmenagogue, phytoestrogenic
SCHISANDRA (*SCHISANDRA CHINENSIS*)	adaptogenic, adrenal tonic, astringent
SESAME SEEDS (*SESAMUM INDICUM*)	phytoestrogenic
SHATAVARI (*ASPARAGUS RACEMOSUS*)	adaptogenic, aphrodisiac
SHIITAKE (*LENTINULA EDODES*)	adaptogenic
SUNFLOWER SEEDS (*HELIANTHUS ANNUUS*)	phytoestrogenic
THYME (*THYMUS VULGARIS*)	astringent
TULSI (*OCIMUM TENUIFLORUM*)	adaptogenic, alterative, antioxidant
TURMERIC (*CURCUMA LONGA*)	alterative, antioxidant, astringent
VITEX (*VITEX AGNUS-CASTUS*)	hormone normalizer
YARROW (*ACHILLEA MILLEFOLIUM*)	antispasmodic, astringent, emmenagogue

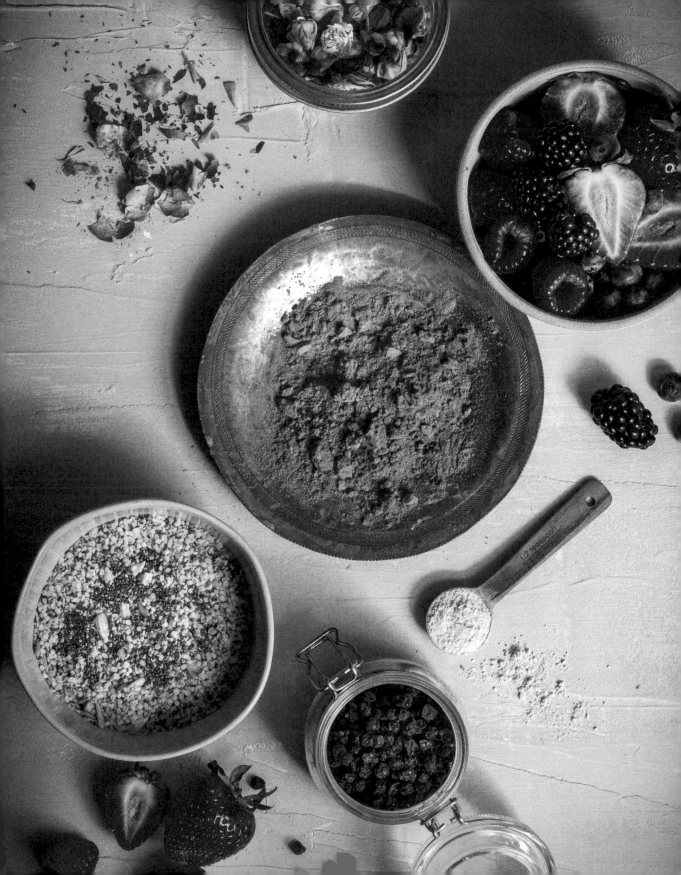

BALANCED BEAUTY BOWL WITH SCHISANDRA

PREP TIME: 10 MINUTES **SERVES** 2

SMOOTHIE BOWL

2 cups coconut water

⅛ teaspoon ground turmeric

1 teaspoon rose powder

1 teaspoon schisandra powder

1 heaping tablespoon plant-based collagen powder

2 teaspoons gelatinized maca powder

3 tablespoons chia seeds

1 frozen banana, peeled

TOPPINGS

½ cup berries (see Note)

2 teaspoons chia seeds

2 teaspoons hemp seeds

1 tablespoon dried culinary-grade rose petals

2 tablespoons unsweetened coconut chips or flakes

An essential way to get a glowing complexion is to nourish and hydrate our bodies with whole foods and herbs that contain anti-inflammatory and antioxidant properties. Berries contain powerful antioxidants called anthocyanins, which give the fruit their richly pigmented color and offer a large range of health benefits, many of which support healthy skin. The herbs in this beauty bowl work together to holistically provide healing qualities needed for healthy cell growth, regeneration, and vibrance.

1. Combine the coconut water, turmeric, rose powder, schisandra powder, collagen powder, and maca in a high-speed blender. Blitz until smooth. Add the chia seeds and banana; blend again until smooth.

2. Pour the smoothie into two bowls and garnish with the toppings in a creative pattern that reflects the beauty of you and your meal.

NOTE: Use berries that are in season and locally available to you in this bowl. Our favorites include strawberries, raspberries, blueberries, and blackberries.

PMS SMOOTHIE

PREP TIME: 5 MINUTES **SERVES** 1

1 cup plant mylk, preferably homemade (page 43)

1 tablespoon raw cacao powder

1 teaspoon reishi powder

1 teaspoon licorice root powder

1 teaspoon vitex powder

½ teaspoon ground cinnamon

2 tablespoons chia seeds

¼ cup almond butter, preferably homemade (page 47)

1 large Medjool date, pitted

1 frozen banana, peeled

1 teaspoon raw cacao nibs, for garnish (see Note)

Although a healthy menstrual cycle would be free from major PMS symptoms, the naturally occurring hormonal fluctuations means there will be moments in our cycle when we need extra TLC, preferably in the form of chocolate. This herbal combination of rich cacao, reishi, licorice root, vitex, and cinnamon gently stabilizes the estrogen and progesterone levels in the body and supports feelings of emotional and physical comfort.

Combine the mylk, cacao powder, reishi, licorice root, vitex, and cinnamon in a blender and process on low speed to combine. Add the chia seeds, almond butter, date, and banana and blend on high for 1 minute, or until smooth. Pour into a glass, sprinkle with the cacao nibs, and serve immediately.

NOTES: Add more almond mylk if you prefer a runny consistency. Add ice if you prefer a colder smoothie.

For an extra-fancy presentation, make a cacao nib rim by dipping the rim of the glass in a shallow bowl of water to wet it, then dipping the rim in a bowl of cacao nibs to coat.

NOURISHING HERBS

VITEX *(VITEX ANGUS-CASTUS)*

Vitex, or chasteberry, the fruit of the chaste tree, is a special herb in Western pharmacology that doesn't have a specific herbal action. Instead, it's referred to as a "hormone normalizer" because it supports the stabilization of estrogen and progesterone levels. It helps to level out the highs and lows in mood and energy around ovulation and menstruation that can destabilize some women.

APPLE OAT SMOOTHIE BOWL

COOK TIME: 10 MINUTES   **SERVES** 1

¼ cup gluten-free rolled oats

1½ apples, cored and chopped

1 Soaked Date (page 48)

1½ teaspoons almond butter, preferably homemade (page 47)

½ teaspoon ground cinnamon

½ teaspoon ground ginger

Pinch of flaky sea salt

1 tablespoon Grain-Free Seed Granola (page 170, optional)

Drizzle of plant mylk, preferably homemade (page 43; optional)

Drizzle of raw honey (optional)

While making this recipe, we did the typical smoothie thing of throwing in tons of ingredients—different spices and herbs, tastes and textures—to make it "interesting." It tasted awful. Heeding our own advice, we got back to basics and kept it simple. All on their own, wholesome oats, apples, a bit of sweet, and a dash of spice taste just right. Remember that you are what you digest, so by taking in this light but nourishing bowl, you will radiate the simple, just-right-ness of you.

1. Combine the oats, apples, date, and 1 cup water in a medium saucepan. Bring to a simmer over medium-low heat, cover, and cook for 8 minutes, or until the apples are very soft.

2. Remove from the heat and purée with an immersion blender until smooth (it's okay if there are a few chunks left).

3. Pour the oats into a bowl and stir in the almond butter, cinnamon, and ginger. Sprinkle with the salt and add granola, mylk, and honey, as desired.

GRAIN-FREE SEED GRANOLA, FOUR WAYS

If you've been reading up on the latest women's health trends, you've probably come across seed cycling. This regimen uses the phytoestrogenic qualities of four different seeds—sesame, sunflower, flax, and pumpkin—to support a woman's natural menstrual cycle. Unlike other holistic remedies that we've discussed in this book, where herbs and foods of opposite qualities are used to balance out the symptoms of a condition, seed cycling matches the energetic properties of seeds with energetic shifts that naturally occur over the course of a month to support natural hormone fluctuations.

There isn't enough scientific evidence behind seed cycling's efficacy; and anyway, to recommend the same hormonal support regimen to all women would go against a foundational premise of this book—that we all have our own unique needs, tastes, and approaches to nutrition. Still, the concept of using seeds to support our hormonal health is a worthwhile one. When we consume seeds, we're accessing the most refined and potent form of nutrition from plants. Seeds are the tiny, beautiful packages in which nature delivers her bounty to us, and a healthy relationship with nature's seeds can bring us closer to our own seeds of creative potential, whether through reproduction or the many other things we pursue in our lives. By eliminating grains, we're also avoiding any potential sensitivities to gluten and wheat (buckwheat and quinoa are both technically seeds), so all their nutrition potential can reach the body's deepest tissues.

Since we are not recommending a strict seed-cycling program, the use of seeds in these granolas is more to incorporate their incredible nutrition and flavors into your mindful eating routine. Sweet and savory varieties make these granolas incredibly versatile for a number of different meals—sprinkled over a smoothie bowl or soup, or straight out of the jar! Store them in the refrigerator or freezer to keep them crisp and fresh all month long. Depending on how you spread the granola over the baking sheet, it may need more or less time in the oven than indicated—be sure to watch so it doesn't burn.

RECIPES FOLLOW

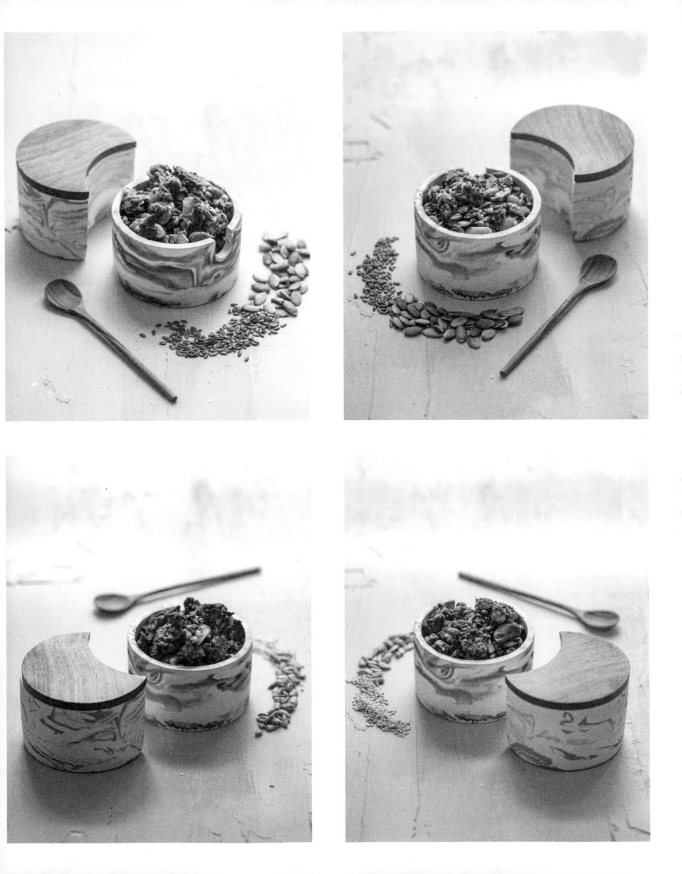

FOLLICULAR PHASE, DAYS 0 TO 13

The follicular stage of the menstrual cycle begins with the start of menstruation and lasts until ovulation. At this time, a good amount of our body's stores of blood, iron, and estrogen have been depleted through the monthly shedding of the endometrium, the lining of the uterus. During the follicular phase (so named because it is when an egg-carrying follicle builds up on an ovary, which will release the egg at ovulation), the body naturally produces more follicle-stimulating hormone (FSH), estrogen, and luteinizing hormone (LH) to support the maturation of the follicle. We thus turn to those seeds with a high level of naturally occurring estrogen—pumpkin and flax. In Ayurveda, we also think of these seeds as more cooling in nature, which additionally supports the production of our cooler, feminine, moon hormones.

SWEET

PREP TIME: 10 MINUTES   **COOK TIME:** 25 TO 30 MINUTES   **MAKES** 4 CUPS

¼ cup chia seeds

¼ cup flax meal

¾ cup raw hulled pumpkin seeds

¾ cup unsweetened coconut flakes

½ cup raw buckwheat groats

2 tablespoons whole fennel seeds

4 teaspoons shatavari powder

1 tablespoon gelatinized maca powder

1 tablespoon coconut oil, melted

¼ cup pure maple syrup

¼ teaspoon sea salt

1. Preheat the oven to 400°F. Line a baking sheet with reusable parchment.

2. Combine the chia, flax, pumpkin seeds, coconut, buckwheat, and fennel in a large bowl. Stir to combine, then add ½ cup warm water. Let sit for 2 to 3 minutes so the chia and flax hydrate.

3. Add the shatavari, maca, coconut oil, maple syrup, and salt. Stir to combine well.

4. Spread the mixture in an even layer over the prepared baking sheet. Bake for 25 to 30 minutes, breaking up the mixture halfway through, until lightly browned but still a little soft. Remove from the oven and let cool for at least 1 hour to crisp up.

5. Break the granola into chunks, then transfer to a large glass jar or airtight container and seal. Store in the refrigerator or freezer for up to 1 month.

SAVORY

PREP TIME: 10 MINUTES   **COOK TIME:** 20 TO 25 MINUTES   **MAKES** 4 CUPS

2 tablespoons flax meal

6 tablespoons warm
  water

1 cup raw hulled
  pumpkin seeds

1 cup quinoa flakes

½ cup slivered blanched
  almonds

½ cup shelled unsalted
  pistachios, chopped

¼ cup chia seeds

2 tablespoons whole
  coriander seeds

2 tablespoons whole
  fennel seeds

1 tablespoon gelatinized
  maca powder

¼ cup plus
  2 tablespoons
  coconut oil, melted

2 teaspoons flaky sea
  salt

1. Preheat the oven to 400°F. Line a baking sheet with reusable parchment.

2. Stir together the flax and warm water in a large bowl and let stand for 5 minutes, or until thickened.

3. Add the pumpkin seeds, quinoa flakes, almonds, pistachios, chia seeds, coriander, fennel, maca, and oil to the bowl with the flax. Stir to combine.

4. Spread the mixture in an even layer over the prepared baking sheet. Bake for 20 to 25 minutes, until golden and fragrant. Remove from the oven. Sprinkle with the flaky salt while still warm, then let cool for at least 1 hour to crisp up.

5. Break the granola into chunks, then transfer to a large glass jar or airtight container and seal. Store in the refrigerator or freezer for up to 1 month.

LUTEAL PHASE, DAYS 14 TO 28

The luteal phase begins with ovulation, or the release of an egg from an ovary. Some women experience a physical sensation with ovulation, and others feel a surge of "heat" that would encourage the egg's fertilization from an eager and available sperm. Biologically, this stage corresponds with a drop in luteinizing hormone (LH) but a building of the corpus luteum (hence the name "luteal" phase). This structure makes progesterone, responsible for gestation and stimulating the uterine lining to prepare for the implantation of a fertilized egg, called a zygote. If a zygote lands in the endometrium, the corpus luteum will keep up the flow of progesterone to prevent contraction of the uterus (which would expel the zygote and you might feel as cramps), as well as estrogen, to maintain the endometrium. If no fertilization occurs, the corpus luteum disintegrates, the endometrium is shed at the end of the luteal phase in menstruation, and the whole process starts again.

Sunflower and sesame seeds, which support progesterone and have warming properties, are what we turn to during the luteal phase. In these granolas, we use tahini, a paste made from ground sesame seeds, which is excellent for all-around reproductive support.

SWEET

PREP TIME: 15 MINUTES   **COOK TIME:** 25 TO 30 MINUTES   **MAKES** 5 CUPS

2 tablespoons flax meal

6 tablespoons warm water

½ cup raw hulled sunflower seeds

½ cup chopped raw walnuts

½ cup chopped or slivered raw almonds

½ cup raw buckwheat groats

1 tablespoon raw cacao powder

1 tablespoon ashwagandha root powder

1 teaspoon ground ginger

1 teaspoon ground cinnamon

¼ teaspoon sea salt

¼ cup tahini, preferably homemade (page 47)

¼ cup pure maple syrup

1. Preheat the oven to 400°F. Line a baking sheet with reusable parchment. Stir together the flax meal and the warm water in a large bowl and let stand for 5 minutes, or until thickened.

2. Add the sunflower seeds, walnuts, almonds, buckwheat, cacao powder, ashwagandha, ginger, cinnamon, and salt to the bowl with the flax and stir to combine. Add the tahini and maple syrup and mix well.

3. Spread the mixture in an even layer over the prepared baking sheet. Bake for 25 to 30 minutes, breaking up the granola halfway through, until lightly browned but still a little soft. Remove from the oven and let cool for at least 1 hour to crisp up.

4. Break the granola into chunks, then transfer to a large glass jar or airtight container and seal. Store in the refrigerator or freezer for up to 1 month.

SAVORY

PREP TIME: 15 MINUTES   **COOK TIME:** 20 TO 25 MINUTES   **MAKES** 4 CUPS

2 tablespoons flax meal

6 tablespoons warm water

1 cup raw hulled sunflower seeds

1 cup chopped raw cashews

1 cup raw buckwheat groats

4 teaspoons whole fennel seeds

1 tablespoon paprika

2 teaspoons dried thyme

2 teaspoons whole cumin seeds

1 teaspoon ground cinnamon

1 teaspoon ground turmeric

Dash of cayenne pepper, to taste

¼ cup tahini, preferably homemade (page 47)

¼ cup extra-virgin olive oil

2 teaspoons flaky sea salt

1. Preheat the oven to 400°F. Line a baking sheet with reusable parchment.

2. Stir together the flax and the warm water in a large bowl and let stand for 5 minutes or until thickened.

3. Add the sunflower seeds, cashews, buckwheat, fennel, paprika, thyme, cumin, cinnamon, turmeric, and cayenne to the bowl with the flax and stir to combine. Add the tahini and olive oil and mix well.

4. Spread the mixture in an even layer over the prepared baking sheet. Bake for 20 to 25 minutes, until golden and fragrant. Remove from the oven. Sprinkle with the flaky salt while still warm, then let cool for at least 1 hour to crisp up.

5. Break the granola into chunks, then transfer to a large glass jar or airtight container and seal. Store the refrigerator or freezer for up to 1 month.

MOON GLOW

LUNAR CYCLES & RITUALS TO CONNECT TO THE DIVINE FEMININE

W omen have been following the patterns of the moon since we've been on this earth as a way to connect to our own divine inner wisdom. The gravitational pull of the moon, and its silvery, cooling light, encourages the quality of *bhrmana*, the Sanskrit word for "heavying," used in Ayurveda, that's responsible for stability, growth, and rest. Its opposite, *langhana*, or bright and energetic energy ruled by the sun, is the favored form of light in our society.

Forming a relationship with the moon is a powerful way to balance the pervasive langhana in our day-to-day lives (which can result in an overflow of stress hormones in the body and diminish the amount of reproductive hormones). These monthly rituals are also beautiful times to engage with nature no matter where you live, and to invite groups of women in your life or community together for reflection and support.

There's no strict formula for conducting a moon ceremony— as long as you're present with your breath and body, you're doing it! The suggestions that follow may help to focus your intention-setting as well as harness the different energy the moon gives off during its twenty-eight-day journey through the sky.

NEW MOON: PLANTING SEEDS OF ABUNDANCE

Plants do their growing in the dark, and as the moon hides her face at the start of the lunar cycle, we're invited to sow seeds of intentions we wish to bear fruit at this moment. They can be long-standing intentions or more immediate ones, and as you imagine those tiny seeds going forth into the dark night, remember the seeds that are inside your body, too—seeds that are ready to grow into any kind of fruit you desire, if you tend them well and lovingly.

For many women, this period also corresponds with the commencement of the menstrual cycle (but if yours doesn't follow this schedule, don't worry!). Enjoy Follicular Seed Granolas (pages 172 to 173), Chicory Root or Rose Cacao (pages 101 and 214), and Milk Thistle & Nettle Tea (page 210) to welcome in this building energy with your food. Consider also incorporating foods and herbs that are nervines, adaptogens, and tonics.

OTHER ACTIVITIES INCLUDE:

- Planting (real) seeds—in an outdoor or windowsill garden
- Self-love oil self-massage (page 215)
- *Supta baddha konasana* (Goddess Pose, page 185) and other restorative yoga postures for the hips
- Grounding & connecting to plant energy (page 135)

FULL MOON: RELEASING UNHELPFUL BELIEFS

A fortnight after the new moon, our female light shines brightest and pulls the waters of the earth toward the shore with height and power all over the planet. We might feel a similar thing happening in our bodies, as ovulation brings a rising tide of hormones and emotions (if your cycle aligns with the moon). At ovulation, you feel strong, vital, and fertile—ripe to conceive, in body and in imagination.

The practice at this time is to remove obstacles that might get in the way of that conception. Maybe they're physical—foods or products that make you feel icky—and maybe they're more about how we go about our lives based on deep-seated systems of personal and social beliefs.

For your full moon ceremony, contemplate ideas or habits that might be hindering your potential to create. Write them down and choose affirmations for clearing and discernment. Choose foods and herbs that are invigorating, aphrodisiac, and warming: Luteal Seed Granolas (pages 174 to 175), Cayenne Cacao with Tahini (page 153), Spicy Turmeric Latte (page 209), and Red Raspberry Leaf & Hibiscus Tea (page 210).

OTHER ACTIVITIES INCLUDE:

- Energizing sun salutations (page 118)
- Moon bathing—stand outside or near a window and let the light of the full moon fall on your face for 5 to 10 minutes.
- Burn sage around your wellness altar, meditation space, kitchen, and bedroom.
- Tidy up your home and pantry, discarding clutter and spoiled foods, to make space for new ones.

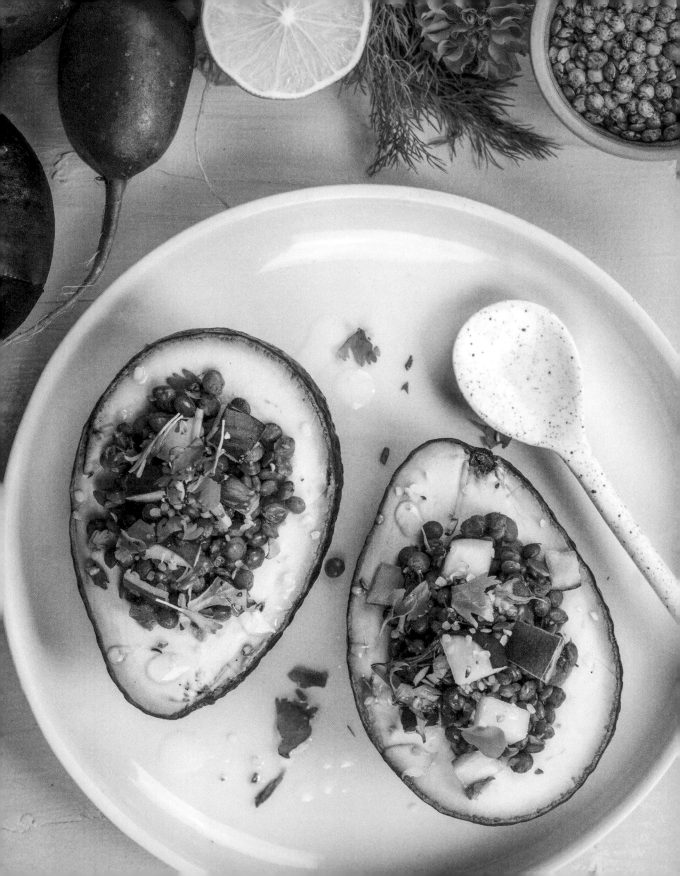

AVOCADO WOMB BOWL

PREP TIME: 15 MINUTES   **COOK TIME:** 20 MINUTES   **SERVES** 1

½ cup dried lentils, rinsed (see Note)

1 teaspoon Herbal Cooking Oil (page 58)

½ teaspoon fresh dill

½ teaspoon ground cumin

½ teaspoon ground nutmeg

½ teaspoon sea salt

1 avocado

OPTIONAL TOPPINGS
Chopped fresh cilantro

Diced red onion

Hemp seeds

Diced radish

Fresh calendula or any edible flowers

Dulse flakes

Fresh lime juice

Herbal Cooking Oil (page 58)

Sea salt and freshly ground black pepper

The womb is the life-force within the feminine. Both a literal and symbolic source of creation, the womb sustains and provides nourishment, just like this recipe. Avocados are enriching, cooling, and soothing, combined with nutritive spices, herbs, and vegetables that tone and provide sustenance when we are needing a connection to our inner wellspring of power. To serve the avocado bowl, you can remove the entire avocado from its skin, making it easier to eat, or leave it in the skin, making it less messy.

1. Fill a small saucepan halfway with 1 cup water and bring it to a boil over high heat. Add the lentils, reduce heat to maintain a simmer, and cook until tender, 20 to 25 minutes. Drain any remaining water from the lentils and return them to the pot. Stir in the oil, dill, cumin, nutmeg, and salt.

2. Halve the avocado and remove the pit. Spoon the lentil mixture into each half. Add desired toppings and serve immediately.

NOTES: We recommend French lentils, because they hold their shape very well without getting too mushy.

SHAKSHUKA WITH PLANT-BASED EGG

PREP TIME: 5 MINUTES   **COOK TIME:** 20 MINUTES   **SERVES** 4

SHAKSHUKA

2 tablespoons Herbal Cooking Oil (page 58)

½ cup diced onion

1 red bell pepper, finely chopped

2 garlic cloves, minced

½ teaspoon ground cumin

½ teaspoon paprika

¼ teaspoon cayenne pepper

¼ teaspoon sea salt

4 large vine tomatoes, quartered

½ cup tomato sauce

1 tablespoon chopped fresh parsley, for garnish

Gluten-free or sourdough bread (see page 130)

PLANT-BASED EGG

½ cup chickpea flour

½ cup vegetable broth or water

2 tablespoons nutritional yeast

1 teaspoon reishi powder

1 teaspoon onion powder

1 teaspoon garlic powder

½ teaspoon ground turmeric

With powerful anti-inflammatory, whole-food, and herbal ingredients, this shakshuka also gives a pinch of heat to awaken the senses and feelings of sluggishness. Pair this dish with any of our coffee substitutes or Lemon Balm Lemonade (page 150) for a blissful breakfast or brunch, preferably in the company of good friends or loved ones.

---

1. Make the shakshuka: Heat the herbal oil in a large skillet over medium heat. Add the onion and bell pepper and sauté until fragrant and the onion is translucent, about 5 minutes. Add the garlic, cumin, paprika, cayenne, salt, tomatoes, and tomato sauce. Reduce the heat to medium-low, cover, and simmer until the mixture thickens, about 15 minutes. Uncover and stir well to break down the tomatoes, then cook the sauce for another 5 minutes to thicken and reduce further.

2. Make the plant-based egg: Whisk together the chickpea flour, broth, nutritional yeast, reishi, onion powder, garlic powder, and turmeric in a large glass measuring jug until well combined; set aside.

3. Use a large spoon to make three wells in the sauce, then divide the egg mixture among the wells. Cover and cook for 3 to 5 minutes, until the egg mixture firms up to your desired texture. You can save the remaining mixture for more plant-based eggs—scrambled or fried! Simply store in an airtight container in the refrigerator for up to 5 days.

4. Remove the shakshuka from the heat, garnish with the parsley, and serve with crispy bread.

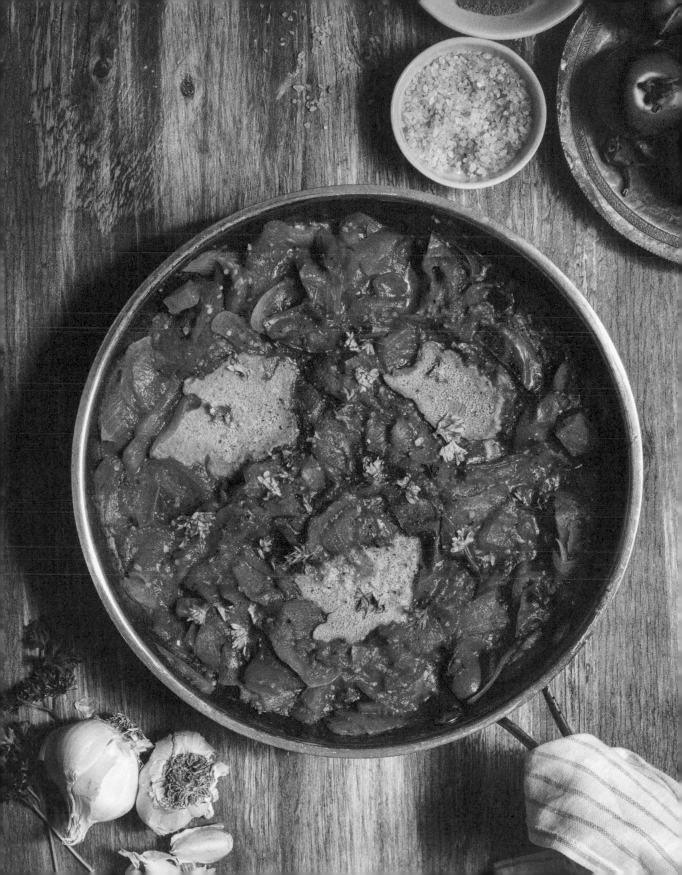

CRUNCHY SEAWEED WRAP

PREP TIME: 30 MINUTES, PLUS 15 MINUTES TO 1 HOUR SOAKING TIME **MAKES** 2 LARGE WRAPS

PICKLED GINGER

1 (1-inch) piece fresh ginger, peeled and thinly sliced

1 tablespoon apple cider vinegar

¼ teaspoon mineral salt (see Note page 82)

MISO-TAHINI SPREAD

½ cup oat pulp (left over from making oat mylk, page 43); or Plain Cashew Cream (page 48)

1 tablespoon white miso paste

1 tablespoon tahini, preferably homemade (page 47)

1½ teaspoons date juice (reserved from making Soaked Dates, page 48)

1 teaspoon grated fresh ginger

½ teaspoon tamari

Juice of ¼ orange

Nori seaweed, which comes in thin sheets, is packed with iodine—an essential nutrient for hormonal health, especially that of the thyroid. While nori may seem frail to touch, it's quite resilient, so don't be afraid of it breaking as you roll. Once you get the hang of the technique, you'll be wrapping up all sorts of things in nori (see the images for the Lemongrass Spring Rolls on page 124 for guidance). You can absolutely swap out the veggie add-ins for others that slice easily—carrots, cucumber, zucchini, even sweet potato—just make sure there is a layer of crunch at the base, so the spread doesn't make the nori too wet. Nori is also delicious flaked into smaller pieces and sprinkled over a variety of dishes.

1. Make the pickled ginger: Combine the ginger, vinegar, and mineral salt in a small jar. Close the jar and shake vigorously for a few seconds. Let rest on the counter for at least 15 minutes or preferably at least 1 hour.

2. Make the miso-tahini spread: Combine the oat pulp, miso, tahini, date juice, ginger, tamari, and orange juice in a medium bowl. Whisk vigorously with a fork until smooth and evenly blended. You should be able to spread it easily, but it should not be liquid or runny. (You will have more spread than you need for this recipe, so store what is left over in a jar in the refrigerator for up to 1 week.)

3. Assemble the wraps: Place a nori sheet on a cutting board or clean work surface with the dull side facing up. Lay down alternating ribbons of jicama and daikon to cover the nori, leaving about one-third of the sheet empty at the top (the side farthest away from you).

4. Add a thin layer of the miso-tahini spread.

5. Add alternating slices of celery and asparagus, and, if using, 2 tablespoons sprouts and 1 tablespoon sesame seeds, if using.

6. Using both hands, begin to roll the filled nori upward, from the edge closest to you to the edge farthest from you. Wet your finger, or use a bit of the extra spread, and use it to "seal" the top section of the nori to the rest of the wrap.

7. Repeat steps 3 to 6 for the second nori sheet.

8. Cut each wrap in half on an angle and serve with a few of the pickled ginger slices alongside. Enjoy immediately.

WRAPS

2 sheets nori

1 cup jicama ribbons (shaved with a vegetable peeler)

1 cup daikon radish ribbons (shaved with a vegetable peeler)

2 celery stalks, thinly sliced

2 to 4 asparagus stalks (depending on thickness), thinly sliced

¼ cup sprouts (fenugreek, alfalfa, or any other variety; see Note; optional)

2 tablespoons white hulled sesame seeds (optional)

NOTE: Sprouting fenugreek seeds is a lovely way to get in the growth mind-set during a new moon or any time of the month, and to try your hand at kitchen gardening. Simply soak 2 to 3 tablespoons of fenugreek seeds in 1 cup water in a large mason jar overnight. In the morning, drain the seeds in a fine-mesh sieve, rinse with cool water, then drain again. Return the seeds to the jar. Set the jar upside down with a small fine-mesh sieve set in the mouth of the jar (so the liquid can run out) in a bowl on your counter, rinsing and draining the seeds twice a day. In 3 to 5 days, you should have a jar of full-grown sprouts, with white tails about 1 inch long. Store them in a covered jar in the refrigerator for up to 1 week, and enjoy as toppings for soups, salads, sandwiches, and grain bowls.

WHITE BEAN BEET HUMMUS

PREP TIME: 10 MINUTES   **COOK TIME:** 1 HOUR   **SERVES** 4 AS A MAIN, 6 TO 8 AS A DIP

2 medium red beets (about 1 cup)

2 garlic cloves, peeled

1 tablespoon extra-virgin olive oil, plus more for garnish

¼ cup tahini, preferably homemade (page 47)

2 tablespoons fresh lemon juice, plus more for serving

1 cup cooked or canned white beans (see page 51, liquid reserved)

2 tablespoons chopped fresh cilantro, plus more for garnish

1 teaspoon ground cumin

½ teaspoon sea salt

Freshly ground black pepper

Whether or not you love pink as much as we do, beets are among the happiest foods we know. They're sweet like candy, filling, and leave their mark on your hands and your pee so you never forget how much you enjoyed them, even days later. Plus, they're incredibly nourishing for your liver and blood (like all red foods), which is helpful during and right after menstruation, in the spring seasonal transition, or any time you're feeling like stress is creating a lot of toxins in your body that needs help being processed. This hummus uses white beans as a base for a creamier texture and a somewhat lighter flavor than chickpeas would give, but if chickpeas are what you've got on hand, they'll work just as well. Just make sure you've cooked your beans really well (see page 51), so they're almost mush. If you hate cilantro, feel free to substitute it for fresh parsley or dill. This recipe makes a modest amount, especially if you eat hummus more like a main than a dip. If I you're serving it for a party, or just want to have more on hand, we recommend doubling the recipe.

---

1. Preheat the oven to 425°F.

2. Cut the beets in half and place them cut-side down on a baking sheet; add the garlic to the pan. Drizzle with the olive oil, cover the pan with aluminum foil, and roast for 45 minutes, or until the beets are very soft when pierced with a knife. Let cool slightly, then chop the beets (if your beets yield more than 1 cup, that's okay, just save them to eat later). Set the garlic aside.

3. Combine the garlic, tahini, and lemon juice in a food processor. Blitz until smooth, about 2 minutes. Add the beets, beans, cilantro, cumin, salt, and a grind or two of pepper. Blitz until well combined, 5 to 8 minutes, adding up to ¼ cup of the reserved liquid or water once the mixture is coarsely chopped, as needed. Taste and adjust the seasoning, adding more lemon juice, cumin, salt, or pepper, as desired.

4. To serve, transfer to a serving bowl and top with additional cilantro, a squeeze of lemon juice, and a drizzle of olive oil, as desired.

SUPPORTED GODDESS POSE

(SUPTA BADDHA KONASANA)

Cultivating a connection with our inner goddess requires a radical act in today's world: slowing down. Restorative yoga is one of the most powerful practices to build up the "muscles" of resting, as the postures are meant to be held for several minutes without any effort of the muscles or bones—the ground, and usually a healthy bunch of yoga props, hold you up, rather than you holding yourself up.

In addition to the postures described in the Gentle Yoga for Relaxation section (page 158), supported Goddess Pose is one restorative yoga posture that not only grounds but also specifically targets the energetic center of reproduction, the second chakra, located at the lower belly between the navel and the pubic bone. It's an area associated with flow and creation, a center of water and abundance. In this posture, the sacrum is situated so all your energy pools toward it, allowing your awareness and *prana*, or life-force energy, to flow down and in, nourishing your deep creative potential.

To practice, fold two blankets or towels into long rectangles and stack them on top of each other lengthwise in the center of your yoga mat. Let there be a slight stair-stagger at the end of the stack closest to you by pulling the top blanket a bit farther back. Take another blanket, fold it in half into a large rectangle, then roll it into a long, skinny roll. Have another blanket or pillow nearby.

Sit on the ground just in front of the folded blanket stack. Bring your feet together to touch and let your knees open out to the sides, making a diamond shape with your legs. Take the rolled blanket and wrap it over the tops of your feet and around your ankles and pull the blanket under and through your lower legs so that it supports your legs completely. Lay back over the blanket stack and fold the extra bit of the top blanket under your head to make a little pillow. The stair-stagger at the bottom of the blanket stack should be filling in the space made by your lower back. Take the extra blanket or pillow and cover yourself, for weight and to stay warm. Rest your arms by your sides or on your belly, palms down. Make any adjustments to the props so you're completely comfortable, without any strain or tension in your joints.

Once you're in the pose, close your eyes and imagine a golden pool at your lower belly being filled with your slow, even breaths. Allow the back of your body to soften into the ground and props beneath you and the front of your body to be protected by the blanket. Rest here for 10 to 15 minutes.

To come out of the pose, remove the props from on top of your body and use your hands on the outside of your thighs to draw your legs up toward each other. Gently roll over to one side and push yourself up off the ground with your hands, letting your head be the last thing to lift. Pause in a seated position and observe your breath, with your eyes closed or looking at the ground, before getting up from the floor.

GOLDEN CREAM OF BEET SOUP

PREP TIME: 20 MINUTES **COOK TIME:** 30 MINUTES **SERVES** 6

2 large golden beets, quartered

1 large yellow onion, halved

1 whole head garlic

1 tablespoon coconut oil

½ cup dried yellow split peas, rinsed

½ cup dried red lentils, rinsed

½ cup almond mylk, preferably homemade (page 43)

¼ cup nutritional yeast

1 teaspoon whole cumin seeds, or ½ teaspoon ground cumin, plus more for garnish

½ teaspoon harissa

¼ teaspoon cayenne pepper (optional)

2 to 4 Soaked Dates (page 48)

Chopped fresh parsley, for garnish

Who doesn't love beets? Roasted, steamed, or puréed, these root vegetables are like rubies from the earth—easily transformed and yet always nutritious and grounding. While red beets usually take center stage, their golden cousins can be a better choice for a number of reasons. They tend to be softer (meaning less cooking time); they stain less (good if you have a white kitchen); and they're a better choice when you're in the second half of your cycle, known as the luteal phase. (But if you make this soup with red beets, it's great during the follicular phase [see page 172], as it supports the generation of new blood during and after menstruation.) Plus, the golden variety affords this soup a plethora of health benefits: their color alone means they have more immune boosters like vitamin C, vitamin A, beta-carotene, potassium, and lycopene. Topaz over rubies? That may not be your preference in gemstone, but when it comes to beets, you're good as gold either way.

Like most soups, this is great for making in big batches to freeze or simply to have leftovers on hand in the days that follow. Add a bit of water or plant mylk when reheating the soup, given its already thick consistency.

1. Preheat the oven to 375°F.

2. Combine the beets and onion in a small baking dish. Slice off the top of the head of garlic to expose the cloves and place it (yes, the *whole* head, with the papery skin) cut-side down in the baking dish. Evenly coat with the coconut oil. Cover the pan with aluminum foil and bake for 30 minutes, or until the beets are soft when pierced with a knife. When the garlic bulb is cool enough to handle, squeeze until the cloves easily pop out of the skins; they should be very soft.

3. Meanwhile, combine the split peas and lentils in a large pot or Dutch oven with 2 cups water. Bring to a boil over high heat, then reduce the heat to maintain a simmer. Cover and cook, stirring every once in a while so they don't stick to the bottom of the pan, for 30 minutes, or until very soft.

4. Add the roasted beets, onion, and garlic, and the mylk, nutritional yeast, cumin, harissa, cayenne, and dates. Stir to combine, then blend with an immersion blender, adding up to ¾ cup water as you go to reach the desired consistency.

5. To serve, ladle the soup into bowls and garnish with the parsley and a sprinkle of cumin (ground or whole seeds), if desired.

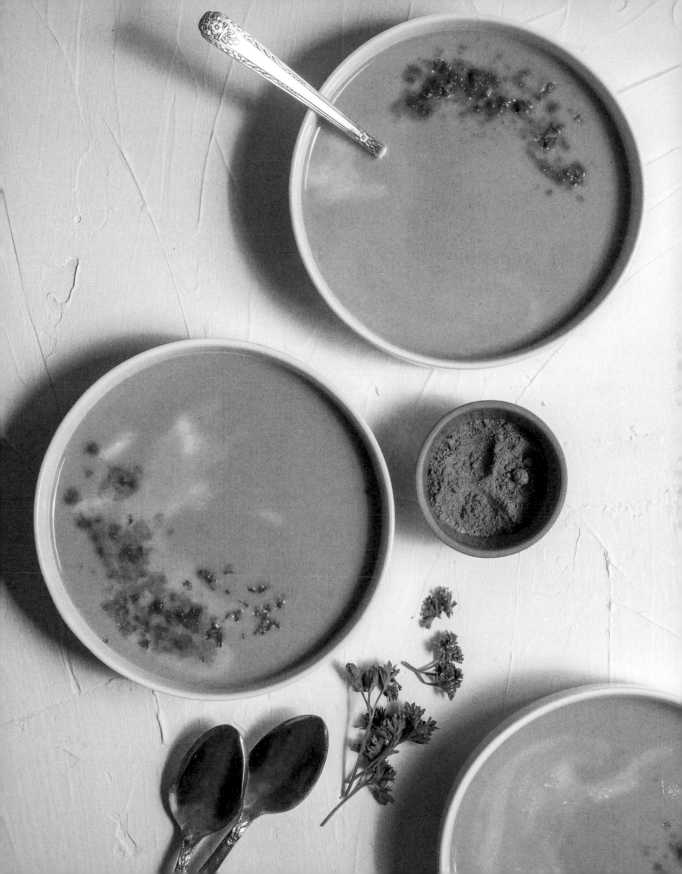

CREAMY BROCCOLI SOUP

PREP TIME: 10 MINUTES **COOK TIME:** 30 MINUTES **SERVES** 6

1 tablespoon extra-virgin olive oil

½ medium white or yellow onion, chopped (1 cup), or 1 leek, rinsed well and chopped (2 cups)

1 garlic clove, minced

2 teaspoons dulse flakes

1 teaspoon dried nettles, plus more for garnish

2 cinnamon sticks

½ cup uncooked quinoa, rinsed

2 cups chopped kale leaves

2 heads broccoli, florets and stems, chopped (5 cups)

1 green apple, cored and chopped

3 cups vegetable broth

Freshly ground black pepper

2 tablespoons oat pulp (left over from making Oat Mylk, page 43), or plain Cashew Cream, page 48), optional

2 tablespoons tahini, preferably homemade (page 47, optional)

While broccoli is not always everyone's friend when it comes to digestion, it is extremely helpful during menstruation. Famous for its nutritional potency, broccoli contains several vitamins and minerals—namely iron, calcium, and vitamins K and C—that synergize to help support a healthy blood supply and strong bones, which need replenishing after our monthly cycle. Turn to this easy, light, flavorful one-pot soup during the first part of your flow, known as the follicular phase (see page 172), to support recovery from your natural detox.

---

1. Heat the olive oil in a large pot or Dutch oven over medium heat for 1 to 2 minutes. Add the onion and garlic, stir to combine, and cook for 5 minutes. Add the dulse, nettles, cinnamon, quinoa, and 3 cups water. Bring to a boil, then reduce the heat to low and simmer for 10 minutes.

2. Add the kale, broccoli, apple, broth, a dash of pepper, and 2 cups more water. Stir to combine, cover, and simmer for 15 minutes, or until the vegetables are soft.

3. Remove from the heat and add 2 cups more water. Blend with an immersion blender until creamy and smooth. Stir in the oat pulp, if desired (it will make the soup creamier).

4. To serve, ladle the soup into bowls and season with additional pepper. If desired, whisk the tahini with a bit of water to thin, then drizzle it over the soup.

ROASTED BRUSSELS SPROUTS, SWEET POTATO & TEMPEH BOWL WITH FENUGREEK DRESSING

PREP TIME: 1 HOUR 20 MINUTES   **COOK TIME:** 30 TO 40 MINUTES   **SERVES** 4 TO 6

MARINATED TEMPEH

¼ cup Herbal Balsamic Vinegar (page 56)

2 tablespoons coconut oil, melted

2 tablespoons tamari

1 teaspoon raw coconut sugar

2 teaspoons whole nigella seeds

2 teaspoons whole fenugreek seeds

Juice of 1 lime

1 (8-ounce) package tempeh, cubed

2 pounds Brussels sprouts, shredded (see Note)

2 tablespoons coconut oil, melted

2 garlic cloves, minced

2 teaspoons paprika

1 teaspoon ground ginger

2 cups cubed sweet potatoes, unpeeled

2 teaspoons ground cinnamon

½ teaspoon ground turmeric

Flaky sea salt and freshly ground black pepper

The Buddha bowl gets an herbal infusion in this sweet and savory, crunchy and chewy dish. Fenugreek tastes cool in the mouth but is beloved for its deceptively heating properties, which help melt away any obstacles creating stagnant elimination but specifically supports cramps, gas, and bloating during menstruation (though it should not be used if you have heavy menstrual bleeding). Seeds give a bit of crunch to the meaty texture of the tempeh—a fermented food, which makes it easier to digest. By shredding the Brussels sprouts instead of simply roasting them whole or in chunks, you get yet another surprising texture that will freshen up any bowl fatigue. While it may seem superfluous to bake all three components on separate baking sheets, doing so gives each ingredient room to roast and harmonize with the spices. It's a small but powerful way to ensure that the integrity of each plant stays strong all the way from your mouth to the deepest layers of nourishment in your reproductive tissue.

1. Make the marinated tempeh: Whisk together the vinegar, coconut oil, tamari, coconut sugar, nigella seeds, fenugreek seeds, and lime juice in a small bowl or shallow dish. Add the tempeh and coat well with the marinade. Let sit for at least 1 hour or up to 4 hours.

2. Meanwhile, preheat the oven to 400°F. Line three baking sheets with reusable parchment.

3. Arrange the shredded Brussels sprouts in a thin layer on one baking sheet. Drizzle with 1 tablespoon of the coconut oil, and toss with the garlic, paprika, and ginger.

4. Arrange the sweet potatoes on a second baking sheet. Drizzle with the remaining 1 tablespoon coconut oil, and toss with the cinnamon and turmeric.

5. Arrange the marinated tempeh on the third baking sheet, reserving the remaining marinade.

6. Place all the baking sheets in the oven and bake for 30 to 40 minutes, tossing the ingredients on each halfway through. The potatoes should be soft when pierced with a fork but browned and crisp on the outside, and the Brussels sprouts should be slightly browning on the edges.

RECIPE CONTINUES

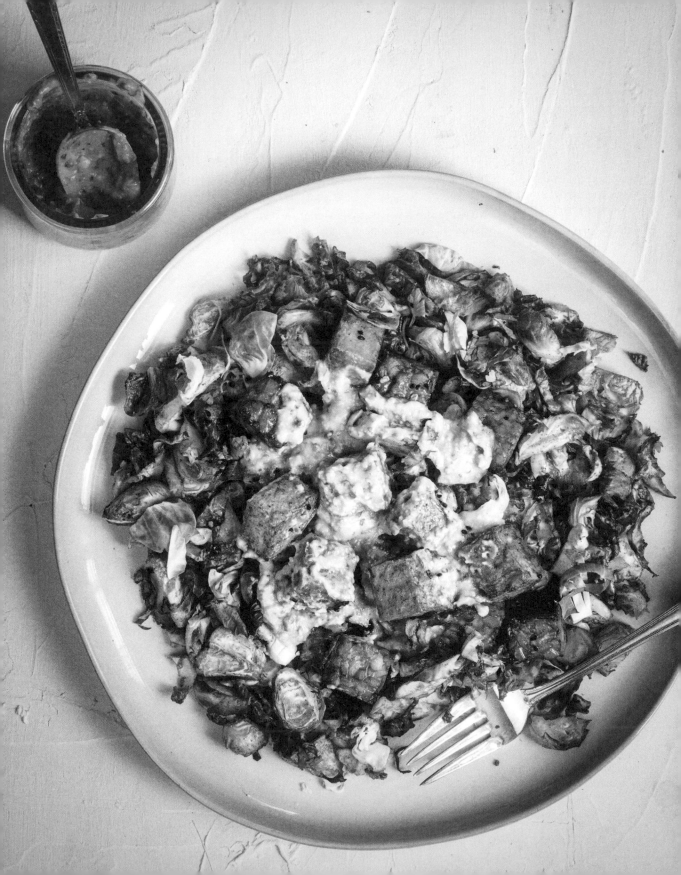

AVOCADO DIP

½ cup chopped avocado (about ½ medium)

½ cup chopped fresh cilantro

1 teaspoon whole cumin seeds, lightly crushed

Juice of ½ lime

7. Meanwhile, make the avocado dip: Combine the avocado, cilantro, cumin, lime juice, and ½ cup water in a medium bowl. Blitz with an immersion blender until smooth and creamy.

8. To serve, layer a scoop of Brussels sprouts, sweet potatoes, and tempeh in each bowl. Drizzle with the reserved balsamic marinade and garnish with a dollop of the avocado dip. Season with salt and pepper, as desired. Store any leftovers in separate containers in the refrigerator for up to 3 days.

NOTE: To shred the Brussels sprouts without destroying your hands, use a mandoline or the slicing blade on your food processor.

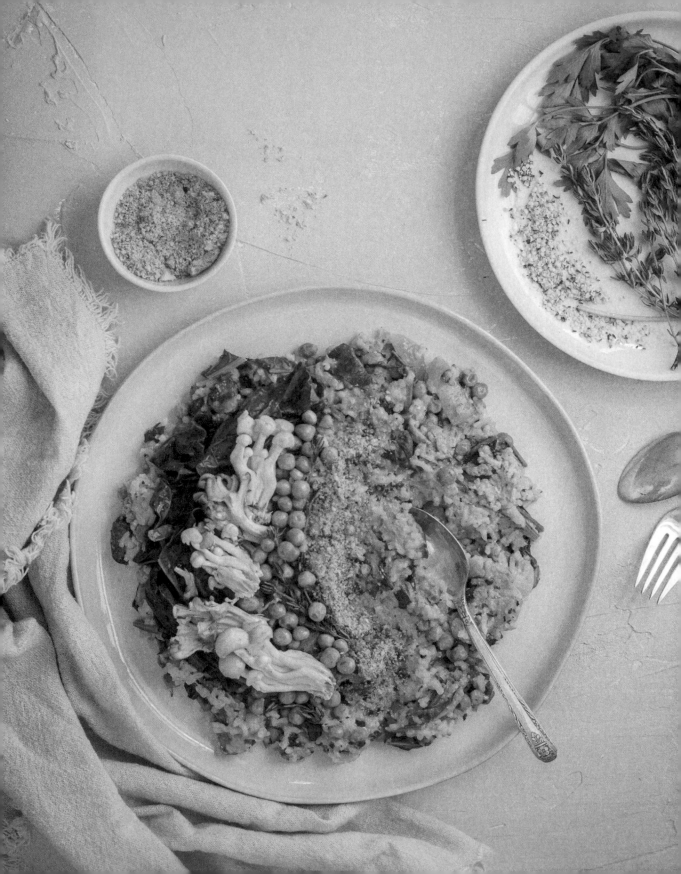

MUSHROOM RISOTTO WITH SPINACH, PEAS & NETTLES

PREP TIME: 5 MINUTES, PLUS 1 HOUR OR OVERNIGHT SOAKING TIME   **COOK TIME:** 50 MINUTES   **SERVES** 8

1¼ cups uncooked white basmati rice, soaked overnight or at least 1 hour

1 ounce dried mushrooms (portobello, shiitake, or oyster)

1 tablespoon dried nettles

2 cups boiling water

3 cups vegetable broth

3 garlic cloves, minced

1 shallot, minced

1 pound white mushrooms, chopped

8 ounces baby bella mushrooms, chopped

⅓ cup rice vinegar

Leaves from 4 or 5 sprigs thyme

¼ cup Plant Parmesan (page 50), plus more for serving if desired

1 bunch spinach, coarsely chopped

10 ounces frozen peas, thawed

Splash of plant mylk, preferably homemade (page 43, optional)

Sea salt and freshly ground black pepper

Fresh parsley, for garnish

This risotto is a savory take on creamy comfort food, as well as being a fresh take on a traditional family meal with a healthy dose of adaptogens. If you've been relying on powdered mushrooms to get in those daily immune-boosters, now's the time to rediscover the power of their original, whole-food form. As you stir, watch closely how the dried mushrooms spring to life. As the steam wafts toward your face, let their aromas harmonize with the umami of the thyme and nettles, another great springtime bitter herb that helps to balance excess moisture. Awareness of the ways foods naturally work together is one of the many small pleasures that making this meal provides.

1. Drain and rinse the rice two or three times, until the water runs clear, then set aside. Set the peas on the counter to thaw.

2. Put the dried mushrooms and the nettles in a medium bowl and add the boiling water. Let sit for 5 to 10 minutes.

3. Pour the broth into a medium saucepan and bring to a boil over medium heat. Reduce the heat to low to maintain a simmer.

4. Combine the garlic, shallot, and 1 tablespoon water in a medium skillet and stir to combine. Cook over medium heat until fragrant and the onion is translucent, about 5 minutes, adding more water if the pan gets too dry.

5. Add the white and baby bella mushrooms to the pan and stir to combine. Cook, stirring frequently, for 5 minutes, then stir in the vinegar and cook for about 5 minutes more, until the mushrooms are soft.

6. Drain the soaked mushrooms through a fine-mesh sieve set over a bowl, reserving the soaking liquid. Add the rehydrated mushrooms and the thyme to the pan and stir to combine. Reduce the heat to low and cover.

7. Add the rice to a large pot or Dutch oven. Add 1 cup of the reserved mushroom soaking liquid, stir well, and bring to a boil over high heat, then reduce to low heat and to simmer, uncovered, until all the liquid has been absorbed. Continue adding the mushroom liquid and then the simmering broth, in 1-cup increments, stirring continuously and letting the rice absorb each addition before adding the next. The rice should be very creamy but still a bit chewy.

RECIPE CONTINUES

8. Remove the risotto from the heat and stir in the plant parmesan. Add the mushrooms, then the spinach and peas. Stir to combine well and let stand until the spinach wilts. (The heat of the pot will wilt the spinach in a few minutes, but lightly covering the pot will expedite the process.) If the mixture got less creamy, stir in a splash of plant mylk.

9. Season with salt and pepper and serve garnished with fresh parsley and more parmesan, as desired.

NOTE: Do your fresh herbs wilt before you get a chance to use them? Revive greens like parsley, basil, and cilantro by giving them a bath in cold water. Simply chop the herbs how you would like to use them, add to a bowl with water, give them a swirl with your hand, and set in the refrigerator until ready to use; you can also store the herbs in the cold water in a container for up to 2 days. The water will perk up wilted leaves, as well as help remove any dirt or debris that a regular rinse in a sieve doesn't catch.

BLISS BITES

When it comes to balancing the nervous system, it's all about dosing—small bites of calm throughout the day can really add up when it comes to leveling the amounts of stimulating and grounding hormones coursing through your veins. There are many ways to microdose on calm—looking out the window, hugging a loved one, listening to a favorite song, taking a walk, and, of course, having a bite of something delicious. When your body and mind are aligned in terms of craving food as comfort, or when you want to have a truly nutritious snack, turn to these sweet treats for a quick mouthful of *rasa*, the Sanskrit word used in Ayurveda for juice, sap, and taste; in other words, the flavor of a blissful and satisfying life. These bites are also quick and fun to make with kids or friends—though make sure you stash enough away for yourself!

MATCHA BITES

PREP TIME: 10 MINUTES, PLUS 2 HOURS FREEZING TIME   **MAKES** 12 BITES

½ cup gluten-free rolled oats

½ cup Soaked Dates (page 48), plus 1 tablespoon date juice

¼ cup almond flour

3 teaspoons matcha powder

½ teaspoon ashwagandha root powder

½ teaspoon ground ginger

2 tablespoons unsweetened coconut flakes

Energize with antioxidant-rich green tea and ashwagandha, both of which support mental clarity without a whole-body spike.

---

1. Combine the oats, dates, date juice, almond flour, 1 teaspoon of the matcha, the ashwagandha, and the ginger in a food processor. Blend until everything is well incorporated and the mixture pulls together, stopping to scrape down the sides as needed.

2. Line a baking sheet with reusable parchment. Place the remaining 2 teaspoons matcha and the coconut flakes in a small bowl. Using your hands or a cookie scooper, form the oat mixture into 1-inch balls. Dust with the matcha-coconut topping. Place the bites on the prepared baking sheet and freeze for at least 2 hours, or until firm to the touch. Store in an airtight container in the freezer for up to 1 week.

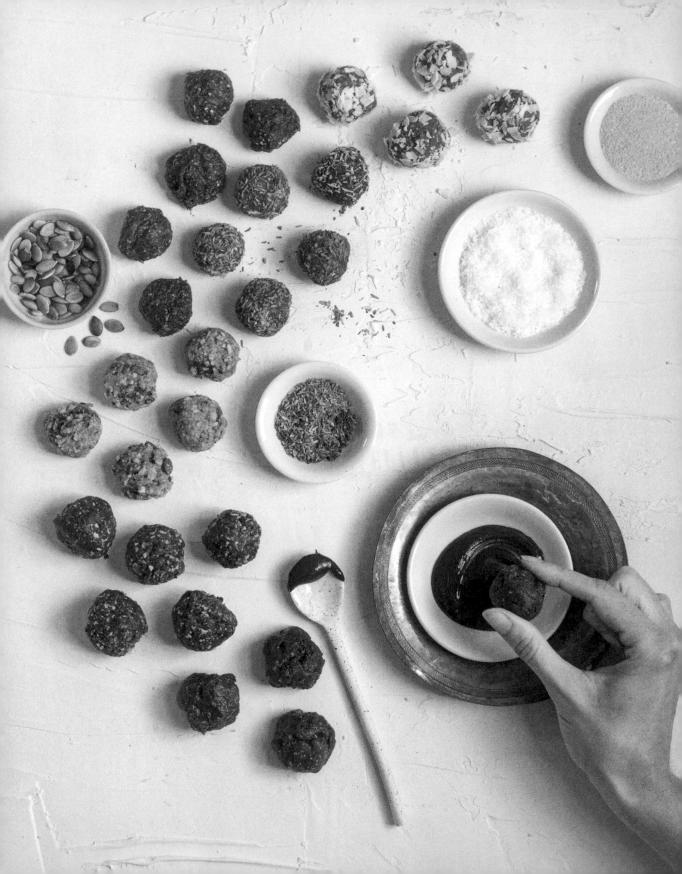

DARK CHOCOLATE FIG OATMEAL BITES

PREP TIME: 10 MINUTES, PLUS 30 MINUTES CHILLING TIME   **MAKES** 18 BITES

2 cups dried figs

1 tablespoon coconut oil, melted

½ teaspoon pure vanilla extract, preferably homemade (page 44)

½ teaspoon shatavari powder

½ cup almond butter, preferably homemade (page 47)

½ cup gluten-free rolled oats

1 cup nondairy dark chocolate chips

Try these bites for a balance of yin and yang—figs, coconut oil, and oats offer cooling and grounding energy; the almond butter and chocolate add a bit of heat; and cacao feeds body and mind with some neurotransmitter happiness.

Combine the figs, coconut oil, and vanilla in a food processor, and blitz to form a coarse paste. Add the shatavari, almond butter, oats, and chocolate chips. Blend until everything is well incorporated and the mixture comes together, stopping to scrape down the sides as needed. Using your hands or a cookie scooper, form the mixture into 1-inch balls. Place the bites in an airtight container, cover, and refrigerate for 20 to 30 minutes, until firm. Store in the freezer for up to 1 week.

COOKIE DOUGH BITES

PREP TIME: 15 MINUTES, PLUS 2 HOURS FREEZING TIME   **MAKES** 12 BITES

¾ cup cooked or canned chickpeas (page 51)

½ cup unsweetened coconut flakes

2 tablespoons raw honey

1 tablespoon almond butter, preferably homemade (page 47)

2 teaspoons gelatinized maca powder

½ teaspoon pure vanilla extract, preferably homemade (page 44)

¼ cup nondairy dark or semi-sweet chocolate chips

Cookie dough isn't just for kids anymore. Aphrodisiac maca turns up the heat of these bites (without needing to turn on the oven) for a bite of grown-up satisfaction.

Line a baking sheet with reusable parchment. Combine the chickpeas, coconut, honey, almond butter, maca, and vanilla in a food processor. Blend until everything is well incorporated and the mixture comes together, stopping to scrape down the sides as needed. Add the chocolate chips and fold in with a spatula or wooden spoon. Using your hands or a cookie scooper, form the mixture into 1-inch balls. Place the bites on the prepared baking sheet and freeze for at least 2 hours, or until firm to the touch. Store in an airtight container in the freezer for up to 1 week.

PUMPKIN SEED CACAO BITES

PREP TIME: 15 MINUTES, PLUS 1 HOUR FREEZING TIME   **MAKES** 24 BITES

1½ cups chopped mixed dried pitted Medjool dates and figs

¼ cup unsweetened coconut flakes

½ cup gluten-free rolled oats

¼ cup pumpkin seed butter, preferably homemade (page 46)

¼ cup raw cacao powder

1 teaspoon ground cinnamon

1 teaspoon ground cardamom

1 teaspoon ashwagandha root powder

Pinch of sea salt

The phytoestrogens in pumpkin seeds help promote hormonal balance during the follicular stage (days 0 to 13) of the menstrual cycle (see page 172). Natural sugar in the fruits and the spot of caffeine in the cacao also make these bites the perfect snack to enjoy after exercising, which is another great way to pull yourself up if your period gets you down.

Line a baking sheet with reusable parchment. Put the dried fruit in a shallow dish and add boiling water to cover. Soak for 10 minutes. Drain, reserving the soaking liquid, and transfer the fruit to a food processor. Add the coconut, oats, pumpkin seed butter, and cacao powder. Blend until everything is well incorporated and the mixture comes together, stopping to scrape down the sides as needed. Add the cinnamon, cardamom, ashwagandha, and salt and pulse to combine well. If the mixture is dry, add some of the reserved soaking liquid 1 tablespoon at a time until it comes together. Using your hands or a cookie scooper, form the mixture into 1-inch balls. Place the bites on the prepared baking sheet and freeze for at least 1 hour, or until set. Store in an airtight container in the freezer for up to 1 week.

MOON GLOW BITES

PREP TIME: 15 MINUTES, PLUS 1 HOUR FREEZING TIME   **MAKES** 10 BITES

¾ cup chopped
  ripe bananas
  (1½ medium), peeled

½ cup unsweetened
  coconut flakes

¼ cup plus
  2 tablespoons
  gluten-free rolled
  oats

2 tablespoons tahini,
  preferably homemade
  (page 47)

5 teaspoons shatavari
  powder

1 teaspoon gelatinized
  maca powder

Make these bites part of your monthly Lunar Rituals (see page 176), with bitter but cooling herbs specific to the female reproductive system, subdued by the clean sweetness of banana and coconut.

1. Line a baking sheet with reusable parchment. Combine the banana, ¼ cup of the coconut, the oats, tahini, shatavari, and maca in a food processor and blend until everything is well incorporated and the mixture comes together, stopping to scrape down the sides as needed.

2. Place the remaining ¼ cup coconut in a small bowl. Using your hands or a cookie scooper, form the oat-coconut mixture into 1-inch balls, then roll them in the coconut to coat. Place the bites on the prepared baking sheet and freeze for at least 1 hour, or until set. Store in an airtight container in the freezer for up to 1 week.

NOURISHING HERBS

SHATAVARI *(ASPARAGUS RACEMOSUS)*

Often paired with ashwagandha in Ayurvedic herbology, shatavari is a cooling herb made from the root of a species of asparagus common to India. Its name means "woman with a hundred husbands" (or "with a hundred roots") in homage to its affinity for the female reproductive system. Although it is excellent for fertility, its adaptogenic qualities mean it can also help ease the transition between stages of life for women and men, as well as support digestion, elimination, respiration, and immunity.

DOUBLE CHOCOLATE BLISS BITES

PREP TIME: 5 MINUTES, PLUS 30 MINUTES FREEZING TIME   **MAKES** 16 BITES

1 cup halved and pitted Medjool dates

1 tablespoon coconut oil, melted

1 ¼ cup nondairy dark chocolate chips

½ cup almond butter, preferably homemade (page 47)

1 teaspoon pure vanilla extract, preferably homemade (page 44)

1 teaspoon ground cinnamon

½ cup unsweetened coconut flakes

If you want chocolate, eat chocolate. These bites are grain-free, allowing the creaminess of the main ingredients to melt right into the chocolate base. Dip 'em twice for a fun truffle layer to seal the deal.

1. Line a baking sheet with reusable parchment. Combine the dates and coconut oil in a food processor. Blend until smooth. Add 1 cup of the chocolate chips, almond butter, vanilla, and cinnamon, and blitz until everything is well incorporated and the mixture comes together, stopping to scrape down the sides as needed. Using your hands or a cookie scooper, form the mixture into 1-inch balls and place them on the prepared baking sheet.

2. For the topping, melt the remaining chocolate in a double boiler. Place the coconut in a small bowl. Dip the top half of a bite into the melted chocolate, then into the coconut. Return to the baking sheet and repeat with the remaining bites. Let the bites set for 10 minutes, then transfer to an airtight container, cover, and refrigerate for at least 30 minutes. Store in the container in the freezer for up to 1 week.

CURATE YOUR OWN WELLNESS ALTAR

A wellness altar is an efficient and beautiful way to gather what you need for *dinacharya*, or Ayurvedic daily practice (see the Root & Nourish Daily Rituals for more, on page 220). Various practices form the container of dinacharya, which helps maintain health and prevent illness when followed regularly. Having a dedicated place in your home for mindfulness encourages a healthy restriction, or "curation," as we prefer to think of it, to minimize distraction and the overwhelming feeling that comes with too many choices. Our altars are places where *bhrmana* (grounding) takes on physical form, so we are reminded to slow down and nourish our inner seeds of creation. They can be the home of your Lunar Rituals (see page 176), the place where you do your daily meditation, or your personal chill-out spot after hectic days or during sleepless nights.

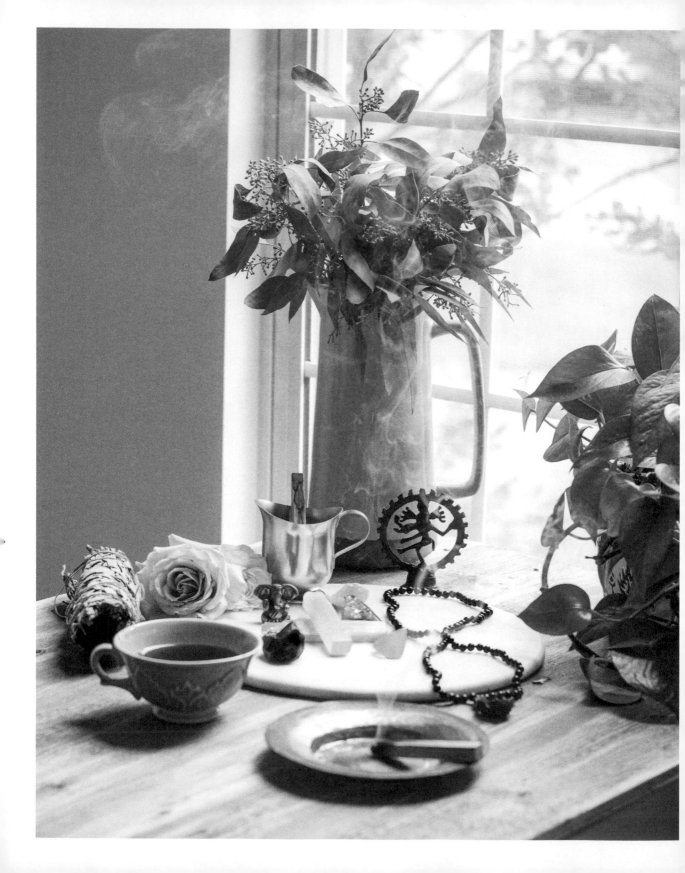

HERE'S HOW YOU CAN CREATE YOUR OWN ALTAR:

SET AN INTENTION: Consider what purpose you want your wellness altar to serve in your life. Are you trying to meditate every morning, make space for a daily home yoga practice, or improve your sleep hygiene? Your intentions will determine where your altar lives but also what it includes, no more and no less, so being clear about what you want your tools to do will help them serve you better.

CHOOSE WHAT SPARKS JOY: In today's world, you could spend thousands of dollars and days of your life trying out all the wellness products available. But more is not better; what works is better. You may read that a certain crystal is perfect for alleviating anxiety, or your friend might tell you about a product that cured her dry skin, but that doesn't mean they'll be right for you. Instead, use your intuition to gather your altar's objects. What feels, smells, and looks beautiful to you? Consider your intention and let the things that will serve that intention find their way to your altar. Having fewer, well-chosen things on your altar will also make it easier to pack them up for travel, so you'll always feel like you're at home. If you need inspiration, choose one item for each of your five senses, as a way to feed yourself with good-quality energy for your practices.

BE ADAPTABLE (AT FIRST): Like routines themselves, your wellness altar might need a breaking-in period. Make it semipermanent at first, so if the location is throwing off your flow, or the objects aren't working for your intention, you can move things around easily. Try not to take these adjustments as signs of failure or that you should give up; rather, consider them opportunities to be creative and curious about things you might not have thought of initially.

BE ADAPTABLE (IN THE LONG RUN): As you settle into your routines and intentions, remember that they might change over time. If, after a few months, your altar needs a makeover, do it! Change is a sign of health, and honoring change will support your pursuit of wholeness and healing. It's less about what you're doing than the act of honoring how you want to feel at any given time, and creating the conditions for that feeling.

You'll know when you've settled on the ideal situation for your altar when coming to it no longer feels like an effort. That's a sign that you've opened a channel to a part of your spirit longing to be nurtured by your rituals, that you and the universe have come into alignment. This is when the wellness altar is no longer a hub for objects serving you, but a place where you can serve yourself—a sanctuary for healing, growth, and discovery; a place to worship within the temple of you.

PEANUT BUTTER LICORICE FUDGE

PREP TIME: 20 MINUTES, PLUS 1 HOUR FREEZING TIME   **MAKES** 25 SQUARES

1 cup full-fat coconut milk

1 tablespoon licorice root

1 teaspoon grated fresh ginger

½ teaspoon Asian ginseng powder

½ teaspoon shatavari powder

3 tablespoons unsweetened coconut flakes or chips

¼ cup raw cacao powder

¼ cup plus 1 tablespoon organic chunky peanut butter

2 tablespoons pure maple syrup

2 pinches of flaky sea salt

Can you count making fudge as baking? We do! Chocolate bliss doesn't need to involve a lot of steps or ingredients, as this simple, wholesome dessert proves. The secret ingredient, licorice root, does a lot of work without overpowering the flavor of the fudge, for those of you who wrinkle your nose at the thought of licorice candy. It's also a demulcent, providing unctuous support and replenishment to reproductive fluids, as well as lending natural sweetness to the fudge. Ginger and ginseng help to balance some of the sweetness and make the heavy, sticky peanut butter a bit easier to digest. This fudge is on the more bitter side, so add more syrup if you prefer a sweeter treat.

1. Combine the coconut milk, licorice root, ginger, ginseng, and shatavari in a small saucepan. Bring to a boil over medium heat, reduce to low, and simmer for 10 minutes, uncovered.

2. Meanwhile, toast the coconut in a dry skillet over low heat for 5 minutes, or until lightly browned. Set aside.

3. Combine the cacao and peanut butter in a medium bowl. Pour the warmed coconut milk through a fine-mesh sieve into the bowl, using the back of a spoon to push out all the liquid. Add the maple syrup. Stir with a heatproof spatula until the chocolate has melted and the mixture is smooth. Taste and adjust for sweetness.

4. Line a small (approximately 7-by-5-inch) glass container with reusable parchment, leaving some parchment overhanging two sides of the container. Pour the mixture into the container and sprinkle the toasted coconut and salt evenly over the top. Chill in the freezer for at least 1 hour until firm to the touch.

5. When ready to cut, lift the fudge from the container using the overhanging parchment and set it on a cutting board. Use a sharp knife to cut the fudge into even squares. Store in an airtight container in the freezer for up to 1 week. Before serving, remove from the freezer for a few minutes to slightly defrost.

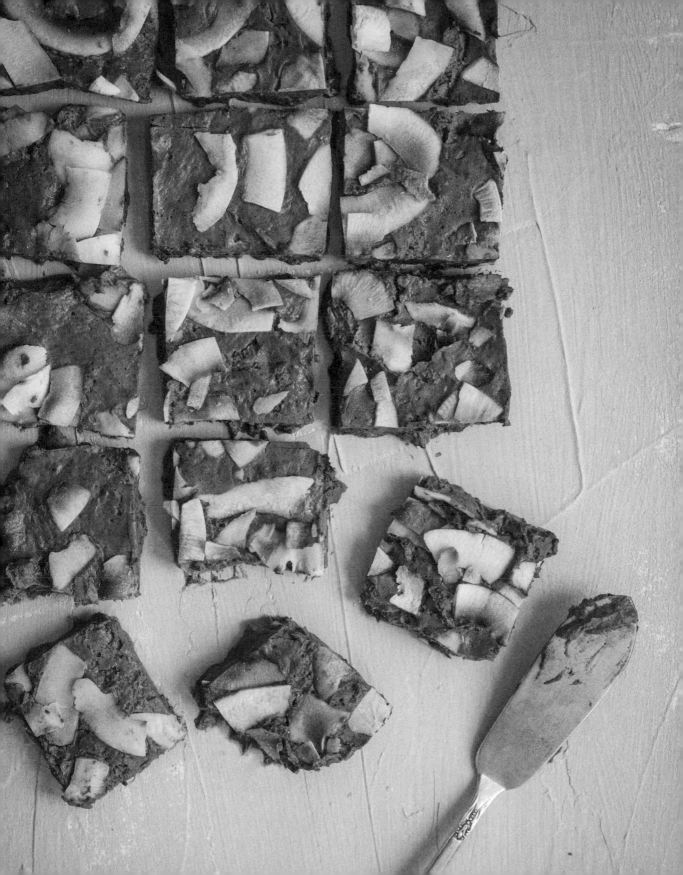

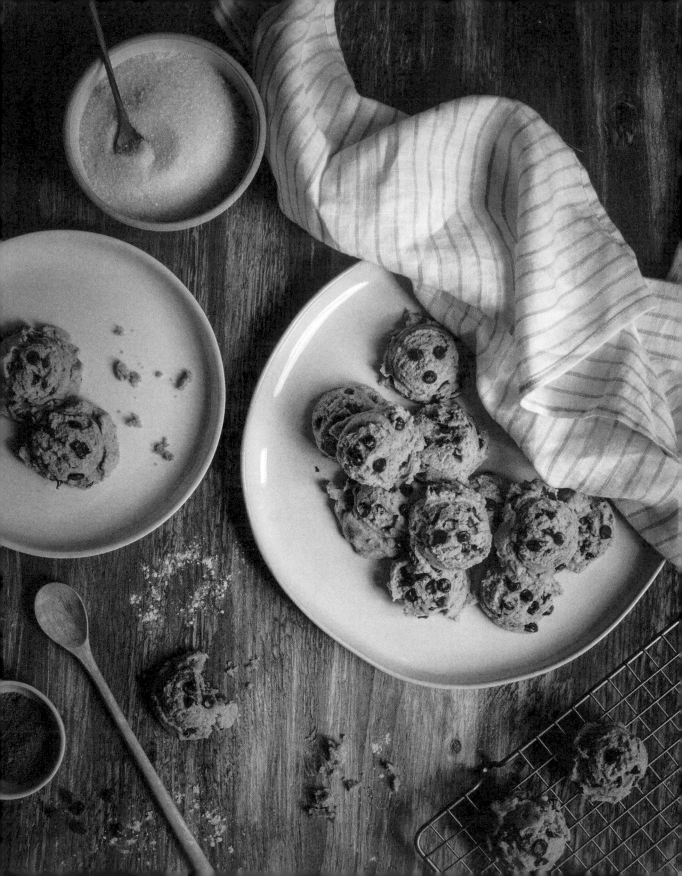

ADAPTOGENIC CHOCOLATE CHIP COOKIES

PREP TIME: 15 MINUTES, PLUS 20 MINUTES CHILLING TIME   **COOK TIME:** 10 MINUTES   **MAKES** 16 COOKIES

½ cup vegan butter
(Miyoko's Creamery
brand preferred), at
room temperature

½ cup coconut sugar

½ cup organic cane
sugar

¼ cup almond
mylk, preferably
homemade (page 43)

2 teaspoons pure vanilla
extract, preferably
homemade (page 44)

1½ cups gluten-free
measure- for-
measure flour blend
(King Arthur brand
preferred)

1 teaspoon shatavari
powder

1 teaspoon reishi
powder

1 teaspoon shiitake
powder

1 teaspoon gelatinized
maca powder

1 teaspoon
ashwagandha root
powder

1 teaspoon baking
powder

¼ teaspoon sea salt

1 cup nondairy dark
chocolate chips

Sometimes the best medicine comes in the form of a classic chocolate chip cookie. And these cookies in particular are packed with adaptogens—feel-good herbs that support the body during times of stress and unease. Combined with dark chocolate, known for its mood-boosting powers, they've become a staple comfort food—and essential medicine—in our homes, especially for mitigating of hormonal highs and lows.

1. Line a baking sheet with reusable parchment.

2. Combine the butter, coconut sugar, and cane sugar in a large bowl and cream together using a handheld mixer or manually with a spatula. Add the mylk and vanilla and mix until creamy.

3. Mix together the flour blend, shatavari, reishi, shiitake, maca, ashwagandha, baking powder, and salt in a small bowl. Add half the flour mixture to the wet ingredients and blend until just combined. Add the rest of the flour mixture, then fold in the chocolate chips. Mix well.

4. Using a small cookie scoop or spoon, place the cookie dough onto the prepared baking sheet 1 inch apart so they have room to spread. Chill them in the freezer for 20 minutes. (This will ensure the cookies keep their shape while baking.)

5. Meanwhile, preheat the oven to 350°F.

6. Bake the cookies for 10 to 12 minutes. Remove from the oven and let cool on the pan for 10 minutes, then transfer the cookies to a wire rack or a plate to cool completely. The cookies will be soft and look slightly underdone, but will firm up to a perfect chewy texture as they cool. Store in an airtight container at room temperature for up to 5 days—if they last that long!

NOTES: You can easily substitute individual adaptogenic powders for a precombined formula, if that is what you have on hand.

   If you need to make the dough ahead of time, simply cover the bowl and refrigerate the dough for up to a day, until you're ready to bake.

TAHINI TRUFFLES

PREP TIME: 10 MINUTES, PLUS 2 HOURS FOR FREEZING   **MAKES:** 12 TRUFFLES

1 cup chopped nondairy dark chocolate (70-80 percent)

1 cup tahini, preferably homemade (page 47)

OPTIONAL TOPPINGS
Ground cinnamon, hemp seeds, and white hulled sesame seeds

Dark chocolate plus sesame tahini is a match made in rejuvenation heaven. Try closing your eyes as you let this bite melt in your mouth and imagine the nourishment coating your nerves with love.

1. Melt the chocolate in a double boiler on the stove. If you don't have a double boiler, you can make one by nesting a bowl with the chocolate inside a pot with a shallow layer of water, allowing the water to boil gently. The water shouldn't touch the bottom of the bowl. Watch the chocolate carefully as it melts to avoid scorching.

2. Pour the chocolate into a glass bowl. Stir in the tahini using a heat-proof spatula. Let the bowl sit until it reaches room temperature, then cover, and freeze the mixture until solid, about 2 hours, or until you're ready to make the truffles.

3. If it's frozen for overnight or longer, let the mixture warm a bit before making the truffles by setting the bowl in the refrigerator until the mixture is scoopable with a spoon.

4. Using your hands or a cookie scooper, form into 1-inch balls. Sprinkle each truffle with the toppings as desired, using a spoon to handle the truffles so they don't melt in your hands. Store in the freezer in an airtight container for up to 1 week.

SPICY TURMERIC LATTE

PREP TIME: 5 MINUTES   **MAKES** 1 GENEROUS MUG

2 cups almond mylk, preferably homemade (page 43)

1 teaspoon ground turmeric

1 teaspoon ashwagandha root powder

1 teaspoon licorice root

½ teaspoon ground cinnamon

¼ teaspoon ground ginger

Pinch of cayenne pepper

1 tablespoon pure maple syrup, to taste

Turmeric lattes may be standard fare on the average coffee bar menu these days, but premade "golden milk" powders might as well be fool's gold. Our latte puts turmeric—the darling of the anti-inflammatory herbs (see Note)—center stage, with a strong supporting cast of herbs with the same properties, plus adaptogenic powers that support the entire system in just the way it needs. On their own, these herbs are very bitter, so add sweetener to suit your taste. For a lighter consistency, use half milk and half water. Make this latte part of your morning ritual, and watch it replace your coffee habit with the first sip. The intentional act of combining the herbs and the rich, grounding qualities of the finished drink will transform any day into golden glory, no matter the weather.

Combine the mylk, turmeric, ashwagandha, licorice root, cinnamon, and ginger in a small saucepan. Raise the heat to medium and bring to a simmer for 5 minutes. Remove from the heat and stir well. Strain the liquid through a fine-mesh sieve into a mug. Stir in the maple syrup and enjoy.

NOTE: You may have heard that adding black pepper is essential when consuming turmeric to enhance the "bioavailability" of curcumin, the active compound in turmeric. Any pungent spice—including the cayenne, ginger, and cinnamon here—will do the same thing, so if pepper's not your thing, don't feel obliged to use it! What's more important is consuming the turmeric in its original whole-plant form, rather than as a curcumin supplement or extract. The other compounds in the whole food are what make turmeric such an effective therapeutic spice, so remember to eat your medicine rather than swallow it as a pill!

CYCLE SUPPORT TEAS

We think of these teas like we do water—simply part of our daily hydration, but with a lot more herbal goodness steeped in. Invest in these herbs in bulk, so you can make a big batch of each blend at the start of the month to last you through your cycle.

MILK THISTLE & NETTLE

COOK TIME: 5 MINUTES   **SERVES** 1

1 teaspoon dried nettle

1 teaspoon milk thistle seeds or powder

For use during the follicular stage (days 0 to 13) of your cycle (see page 172), with bitter herbs to support the liver and reduce inflammation. Milk thistle also has properties that mimic estrogen in the body so as to replenish that hormone after its natural decline during menstruation. It also may stimulate breast milk production and bring on missing or irregular periods.

RED RASPBERRY LEAF & HIBISCUS

COOK TIME: 5 MINUTES   **SERVES** 1

1 teaspoon dried red raspberry leaf

1 teaspoon dried hibiscus flowers or hibiscus powder

For the luteal stage (days 14 to 28) of your cycle (see page 174), this tea uses herbs that tonify the uterus, can stimulate menstrual flow, and can support heavy bleeding and cramps. Both herbs are also great for the skin, augmenting the natural glow that arrives during the second half of the menstrual cycle, when estrogen levels are highest.

Bring 2 cups of water to a boil in a small saucepan or tea kettle. Place the herbs in a tea infuser or strainer, then place the infuser in a mug (or set the strainer on top). Pour the water over, and steep for 5 minutes. Enjoy warm.

TEATIME ANYTIME

Want to make sure you can have a cup of calm anytime? Prepare your own loose-leaf herbal tea blends in bulk. Simply combine equal amounts of dried herbs (¼ cup to 1 cup of each) in a glass jar, mix well, and seal; store in a cool, dark place, up to 6 months. Use 1 to 2 teaspoons of the tea blend per serving. Use this method for any of the loose-leaf teas or spice blends in this book.

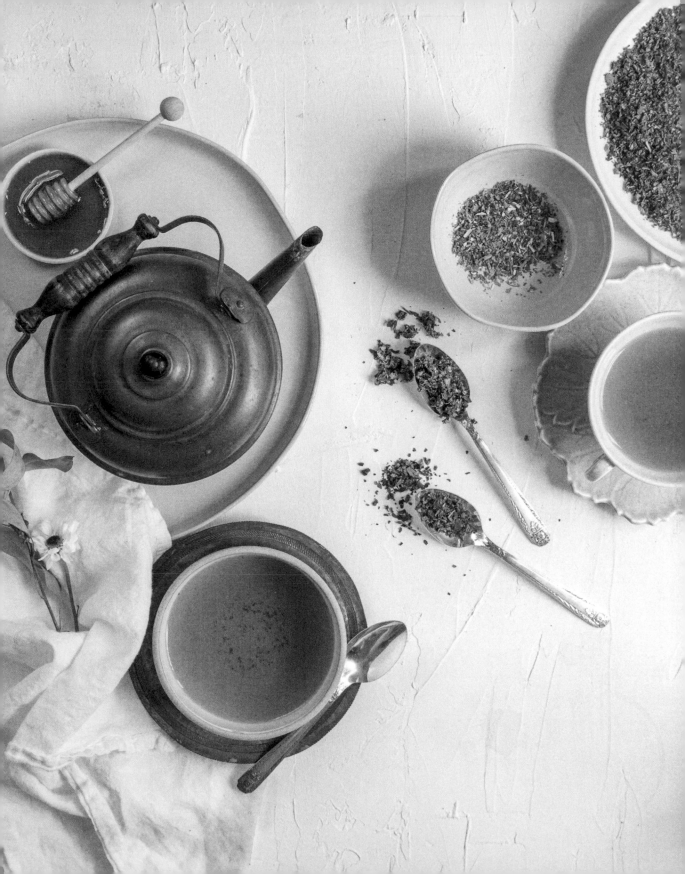

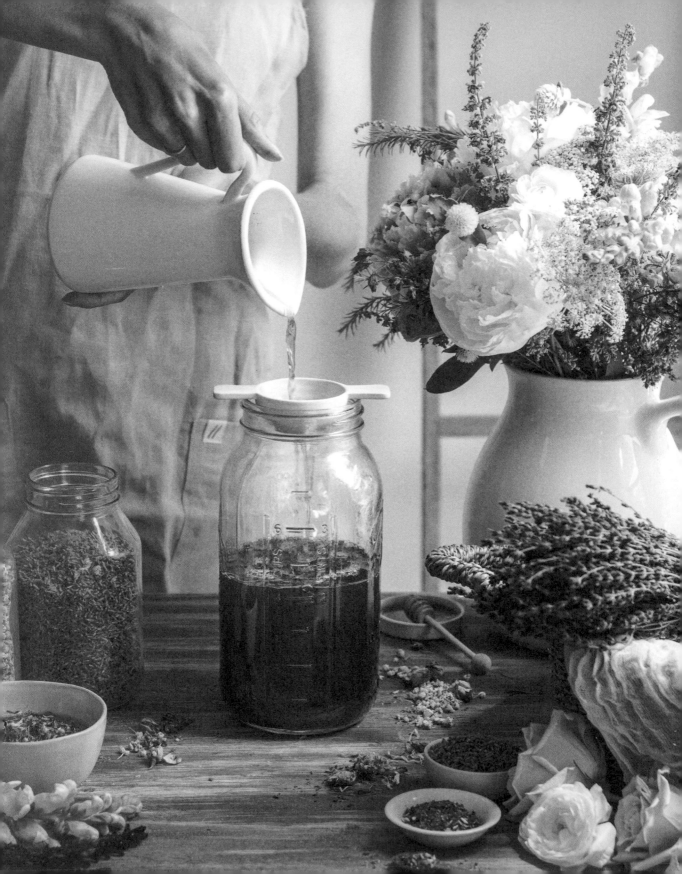

GARDEN GODDESS TONIC

PREP TIME: 5 MINUTES, PLUS 25 MINUTES STEEPING TIME   **SERVES** 4

1 tablespoon dried red raspberry leaf

1 tablespoon dried calendula flowers

1 tablespoon dried chamomile flowers

2 teaspoons dried nettle

2 teaspoons dried culinary-grade rose petals

2 teaspoons dried meadowsweet

2 teaspoons dried skullcap

1 teaspoon dried motherwort

1 teaspoon raw honey or sweetener, to serve (optional)

These beautiful herbs and flowers, even in their dried form, come together in a powerful formula to create a tonifying effect throughout the reproductive system and the body as a whole. Drink a cup of this goddess tonic each day to experience the synergy of feminine herbal energy and cultivate a deeper sense of wellness and connection to the divine within you. If you have the fresh herbs and flowers on hand, feel free to use them as an additional natural (and beautifying!) garnish for your tea.

1. Fill a large pot with 4 cups water and bring it to a rolling boil over high heat. Add in the herbs, cover, and reduce the heat to maintain a low simmer. Let steep for 25 minutes to extract the tonifying herbal properties.

2. Strain the liquid into a large jar. Let cool, seal, and store in the refrigerator for up to 3 days, drinking 1 to 2 cups of the tonic, chilled or at room temperature, per day.

NOTES: Unlike other teas and drinks in this book, the Garden Goddess Tonic has more of a medicinal potency thanks to the longer steeping time of the herbs. The taste is more bitter as a result, making it the kind of drink you take down in one go rather than sip leisurely. If the bitterness is too much for you, go ahead and add some honey or your preferred sweetener when you drink it (but not to the entire batch).

Use the steeped herbs as compost to keep the life cycle of the herbal energy flowing in a sustainable way.

NOURISHING HERBS

CHAMOMILE *(MATRICARIA RECUTITA)*

Chamomile is a wonderfully versatile herb that has been used for centuries because of its wide range of actions and medicinal properties. German chamomile is the most widely used in plant medicine. An annual that can grow up to 24 inches, chamomile is native to Europe, North Africa, and parts of Asia. Both the flowers and the leaves are edible, although they have a different taste, and can be described as slightly bitter, sweet, and aromatic. The dried flowers are most commonly used in teas and herbal preparations.

Chamomile is a mild nervous system sedative, antispasmodic, anti-inflammatory, antiseptic, carminative, antimicrobial, and vulnerary. It is used medicinally to support frayed nerves and provide a sense of calm, and it can pacify an upset stomach or digestive unrest, support muscle spasms, and soothe the skin.

The genus name *Matricaria* is rooted in the Latin word *matrix*, which means "womb," hinting at its beneficial effects for women.

ROSE CACAO

COOK TIME: 10 MINUTES **SERVES** 1 GENEROUS CUP

2 tablespoons raw cacao powder

½ teaspoon gelatinized maca powder

½ teaspoon ashwagandha root powder

½ teaspoon shatavari powder

1 cinnamon stick

¼ cup full-fat coconut milk

½ teaspoon rose powder

1 teaspoon raw honey

1 teaspoon lightly crushed dried culinary-grade rose petals

In case you haven't guessed yet, we were really inspired by pink in this section. Gender norms aside, the color pink is associated with the heart chakra in yoga—the energetic center related to communication and love. This delicately sweet yet indulgent drink is one of our favorite ways to nourish our hearts at the deepest level of body, mind, and spirit. Cacao restores vital minerals and antioxidants that may be lost during menstruation, and is a mood-lifter and calming to the nervous system. Ayurvedic herbs ashwagandha and shatavari act with special potency as an aphrodisiac and tonic on the reproductive tissues. All together, this pretty cacao allows your inner radiance to shine in all its vibrant colors.

1. Mix the cacao, maca, ashwagandha, shatavari, and ½ cup water in a small saucepan until smooth. Add 1½ cups more water, the cinnamon stick, and the coconut milk and bring to a boil over medium heat. Reduce the heat to low, cover, and simmer for 8 minutes.

2. Remove from the heat and whisk briskly with a fork or an electric frother.

3. Let cool to the temperature you would like to drink it, then stir in the rose powder and honey. Garnish with the crushed rose petals.

NOURISHING HERBS

ROSE (ROSA DAMASCENA)

Rose has been used and valued for its beauty and aromatic qualities for thousands of years. It is known for its energetic ability to open the heart, which in Ayurveda, traditional Chinese medicine (TCM), and Unani (Greek-Arabic) medicine traditions, is believed to be both a physical organ and the seat of consciousness, giving support to our perceptions of the world around us. These schools teach that the rose has a powerful effect on our emotions and spiritual health.

The part of the rose plant used most often in herbal cooking is the rose petals, which are dried and used whole or ground into a powder. Rose hips are used as well, but they have a distinctive flavor (different from rose petals). Its herbal actions are used medicinally as a gentle sedative, nervine, gentle astringent, nutritive, tonic, antispasmodic, aphrodisiac, anti-inflammatory, and antimicrobial.

SELF-LOVE
SELF-MASSAGE
(ABHYANGA)

One way to root and nourish a depleted nervous system is through the sense of touch, particularly self-massage. Unlike having someone else massage you, which certainly has its time and place, self-massage supports a more compassionate relationship with our bodies, a better understanding of their terrain and their tendencies, and a feeling of empowerment as we heal ourselves with our own hands.

In Ayurveda, self-massage is typically done with oil in a ritual called *abhyanga*. (A synonym is *snehana*, the word for "oil," which also translates to "mother's love.") To practice, lay a towel on the floor in a warm bathroom to sit on; don't use your favorite towel, since it will probably get some oil on it. Warm ½ cup oil (see list below) in a glass jar set inside a bowl with boiling water. Apply the oil all over your body from feet to head, spending up to 5 minutes on each major body part. Use long, even strokes over your limbs and clockwise circular motions over your joints, sacrum, hips, belly, chest, scalp, and ears. Apply very gentle pressure, since this is less deep-tissue work and more about coating the body with a feeling of safety and nourishment. Let the oil soak in for 5 to 10 minutes, then (carefully) step into the shower and rinse off the oil with hot water—without soap. The oil acts as a cleanser to remove any dirt and oil naturally produced by the skin. (You can shampoo your hair if you oiled your head, and you may find you need to wash it twice to get all the oil out; washing your underarms, pelvic region, and feet with soap is also fine.)

Enjoy longer abhyangas once a week or once a month (or tie them to your Lunar Rituals, page 176), and quickie versions daily, with less oil and less time, when you shower in the morning or at night. To find the oil that's right for you, use the guide below.

DRY, COLD SKIN (OR FALL SEASON): Sesame, jojoba, or almond oil

DAMP, COLD SKIN (OR SPRING SEASON): Sesame, mustard, or almond oil

OILY, HOT SKIN (OR SUMMER SEASON): Coconut, sunflower, or olive oil

You can enhance your abhyanga experience by lighting candles, listening to calming music, and decorating your space with serene items from your Wellness Altar (page 201). Regular abhyanga will not only support your nerves, but can also support healthy digestion and elimination, sleep, complexion, overall body tone, and menstruation.

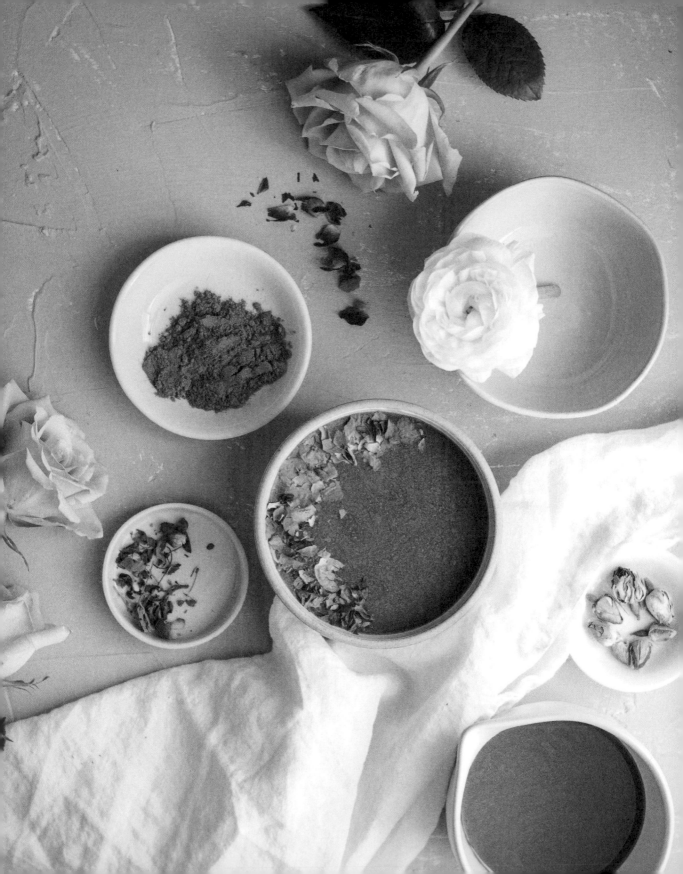

PINK MOON MYLK

PREP TIME: 5 MINUTES   **COOK TIME:** 10 MINUTES   **SERVES** 1

1½ cups almond mylk, preferably homemade (page 43)

1 teaspoon licorice root

1 teaspoon dried red raspberry leaf

1 teaspoon dried tulsi

1 teaspoon rose powder

½ teaspoon hibiscus powder

1 teaspoon raw honey or other sweetener, or to taste (optional)

The macrocosmic cycles of nature—the waxing and waning of the moon, the ebb and flow of the tides, and the changes of the seasons—are reflected on a smaller scale in the menstrual cycle of the individual female body. This Pink Moon Mylk is a wonderful support to the various phases through which we move, symbolically in its color, and within the properties that this combination of herbs holds. It assists in uplifting your mood, contains antispasmodic and anti-inflammatory qualities, and is an aphrodisiac. It also helps regulate menstruation and has uterine-tonifying properties to support you at any phase in your monthly cycle. Enjoy it as part of your Lunar Rituals (page 176), or any time you are looking for the feeling of a warm hug in a cup.

1. Combine the mylk, licorice root, raspberry leaf, and tulsi in a small saucepan. Bring to a gentle boil over medium heat, reduce the heat to low, cover, and simmer for 10 minutes.

2. Strain the liquid through a fine-mesh sieve into a mug. Add the rose and hibiscus powders and whisk briskly by hand or with an electric frother, until well combined. Let cool to the temperature you would like to drink it, then stir in the honey, if desired.

TULSI (OCIMUM TENUIFLORUM)

NOURISHING HERBS

Tulsi is one of the most revered plants in herbal medicine and is thought of in Ayurveda as a goddess incarnated as a plant—hence its other common name, Holy Basil. Its medicinal and spiritual properties are infinite, including as a lung tonic, adaptogen, immune supporter, complexion enhancer, and more. While there are many varieties of tulsi, Rama tulsi (Ocimum tenuiflorum) is the most popular and accessible and has more cooling properties that support female energetics. Among its many names is "the queen of herbs," making it a great addition to the ways you support your feminine energy. Drinking a cup of tulsi tea, either as part of this Pink Moon Mylk or on its own, is a helpful way to support longevity, immunity, respiration, and everyday balance in mind, body, and spirit.

OJAS MYLK

PREP TIME: OVERNIGHT SOAKING   **COOK TIME:** 12 MINUTES   **MAKES** 1 GENEROUS MUG

1 cup almond mylk,
    preferably homemade
    (page 43)

1 or 2 Soaked Dates
    (page 48)

8 whole raw almonds,
    soaked overnight and
    peeled

¼ teaspoon ground
    turmeric

¼ teaspoon ground
    ginger

¼ teaspoon ground
    cardamom

¼ teaspoon ground
    cinnamon

Sometimes the deepest nourishment comes in the humblest of packages. This highly rejuvenating drink is one of Ayurveda's finest medicines, a combination of simple but potent ingredients that get refined into the vital substance known as ojas at the core of our immunity and vitality. Drink ojas mylk in the morning as a light breakfast or at night as a light dinner or evening tonic; if drinking it at night, replace the ground ginger with ground nutmeg to promote sleep. For a richer version, use all mylk or less water.

Combine the mylk, dates, almonds, turmeric, ginger, cardamom, cinnamon, and 1 cup water in a medium saucepan. Bring to a boil over medium-high heat, then reduce the heat to maintain a simmer. Cover and cook for 10 minutes. Remove from the heat and blend with an immersion blender until frothy and smooth. Pour into a mug and enjoy.

YOUR OJAS
IS GLOWING

Ayurveda identifies a substance in the body called *ojas,* which is described as silvery and viscous, coating the body's internal surfaces with immunity, vigor, and a moonlike glow. We all have a specific quantity of ojas when we're born, and it can be depleted by activities like overwork, not sleeping, toxic relationships, and eating poor-quality foods. The good news is, you can also replenish your ojas by taking care of your digestive system, since so much of our immunity is based on the health of our microbiome.

You see, according to Ayurveda, ojas is the end product of a thirty-five-day, seven-layer digestive process, wherein an apple you eat on the first of the month will make its way through the body all the way to the deepest layer, the reproductive tissue, by the end of the month, at which point that apple has been refined into its purest essence—this is ojas. What and how we eat, therefore, is directly correlated to the quality and quantity of ojas in our body.

According to Ayurvedic texts, dates, soaked almonds, kitchari (page 81), spiced milk, high-quality fats, sesame and tahini (page 47), and cooked organic vegetables support ojas, but all the recipes in this book—especially the cacao drinks on pages 101, 153, 215, and the Spicy Turmeric Latte on page 209—provide ojas-building nourishment in their own way. Remember what you eat is only as good as what you digest, so feeding yourself with plenty of undisrupted sleep, good company, nature, and beautiful sounds, sights, smells, colors, and tastes to keep your digestion strong will also keep you glowing with ojas.

ROOT & NOURISH— DAILY RITUALS

Now that you know the many, many ways you can incorporate herbs into your daily life, it's time to start to curate daily rituals for your ongoing well-being. In Ayurveda, the practice of daily self-care is called *dinacharya*, and incorporates a number of cleansing, mindfulness, and nourishing practices that are suited to an individual's current state and long-term constitution. The suggestions we provide in this section are meant to be a template for creating your own dinacharya, using herbs in all five pillars of health, which you should customize to suit your needs.

NUTRITION

You know by now that eating is not just about getting calories and nutrients to fuel your body. Consuming food is a sacred act, one in which the miracle of your body performs an amazing feat of incorporating and transforming something from nature into you. As you plan and prepare your meals, consider your needs for the day (energetic, nutrition, tastes, cravings), as well as any long-term conditions or imbalances you are working with. Keeping in mind the Rule of Threes for Rooted Digestion (page 72), a general schedule for eating might look like the following column. Don't forget the principles of mindful eating to ensure your body gets all the nutrition of your herb-ful meals!

6 A.M.: Wake up, Cooked Water with Lemon (page 97), Ayurvedic CCF Tea (page 98), or another herbal digestive tea

8 TO 9 A.M.: Breakfast—make it warm and cooked, light in texture, but dense enough to carry you through to lunch without snacking.

12 TO 1 P.M.: Lunch—make it your biggest meal, to take advantage of the sun's fiery energy outside to aid your internal digestive fire (known as *agni* in Ayurveda). Cooked food is still preferable, but lunch is the time for anything raw, including smoothies, since your digestion will be stronger at midday.

3 TO 4 P.M.: Afternoon refresh—many people experience the 3 p.m. slump, reaching for caffeine or snacks to boost their energy during this time of day when the mind can feel scattered and attention shrinks. Instead, make a ritual out of your afternoon herbal tonic or tea. Step away from what you're doing to prepare the drink and wait for it to steep, letting the aromatic steam waft toward your face. If you are genuinely hungry, or won't be eating dinner until late, try one of the milky teas on pages 152 and 153), or choose a Bliss Bite (page 195) or a whole piece of fruit for a snack. If you're not hungry but have an appetite for some sensation, take a sense break with mindful breathing, a walk around the block, or a gentle stretch, or just look out the window. The nourishment you get from these practices will feed you with *prana*, or life-force energy.

5 TO 6 P.M.: Dinner—a light, cooked dinner may not be what the Western culture promotes, but it allows for easier digestion (since your body doesn't need a lot of fuel at the end of the day) and sounder sleep. If you're having digestive issues, avoid raw foods (including salad and raw fruits as dessert), which are harder to digest.

8 TO 9 P.M.: Evening tonic—a grounding, warming drink can be a great way to prepare yourself for sleep, which is also the time when many rejuvenating herbs (like ashwagandha and shatavari) can be more easily assimilated by the body. It's also a wonderful substitute for the traditional dessert, if your body is telling you it needs a different type of nourishment. Try to leave at least 1 hour between finishing your tonic and going to bed, to avoid waking up during the night to use the bathroom.

REST & SLEEP

We cannot function without sleep. Period. You know this, we know this, and yet the temptation to resist sleep is ingrained in us from the time we're children, making a fuss before bedtime. By creating healthy sleep rituals, you can prepare the body and mind for the important work that it does in the night—cleansing, detoxifying, and repairing—and maybe even start to look forward to sleep as more than just an antidote to exhaustion.

From a digestive standpoint, the best way to ensure restful sleep is to give your gut some space. Refrain from eating large, heavy meals at night, which will give your body too much work to do once your head hits the pillow. The relaxing teas found throughout this book (Creamy Chai Latte, page 152; and Lavender, Chamomile & Rose Tea, page 157; Herbal Lullaby, page 159; Pink Moon

Mylk, page 217) can help support a transition into a parasympathetic state, so the mind is not racing as you move toward rest.

Other rituals that can support sleep include turning off your devices 1 to 2 hours before bed, restorative yoga and breathing practices (pages 143 and 158), sleep-promoting essential oils like lavender and vetiver, and *abhyanga* (page 215) on your whole body or the soles of your feet (which draws energy down from the head).

MOVEMENT

Our bodies evolved to move, and regular movement is essential to smooth digestion, a robust immune system, and sound sleep. Yet our society increasingly demands that we spend more time in one place, sitting in front of devices for work or pleasure (and that huge gray area in between). There are many trackers, apps, and programs that can remind you to move throughout the day, and even give motivational goals; if those serve you, then by all means do what works for your schedule and personality. Making movement organic and enjoyable, though, will be the surefire way to ensure you do it! If going to the gym or running feels oppressive to you, find something else that's more your jam—maybe it's yoga, maybe it's having dance parties in your kitchen while you cook (but not while eating).

When carving out space in your day for movement, consider the other responsibilities your body has in terms of digestion and sleep. Ideally, movement happens between 6 and 10 A.M. or P.M., when the internal and external environment is a little more grounded and heavy, thus able to maintain the endurance needed for exercise. As a general rule, move before you eat (rather than after), with the exception of a gentle walk after a meal to encourage the downward movement of food through your GI tract (page 79); but don't exercise when you're actively hungry! When you're hungry, you should eat.

Morning movement can be more vigorous, especially if you're feeling sluggish in body or mind (try the Belly Yoga on page 79 or Energizing Sun Salutations on page 118), but keep any movement in the evening on the gentler side so as to not put your nervous system into high gear before you sleep (check out the Gentle Yoga for Relaxation on page 158). Aside from deliberate exercise, make movement part of how you live. Stretch, jump, play, dance, roll around on the floor—all these things tap into the natural instincts of your animal body, which connect you more deeply to the natural world.

Remember, too, that a body in motion needs fuel! So be sure that if you are intentionally increasing your movement or just moving more than usual, notice how it affects your hunger, digestion, and elimination, and adjust accordingly. Hydrate properly, too—try the Herbal Waters on page 54.

CONNECTION

Connection is essential to our physical and mental health. Humans are social creatures and making time to be in the company of compassionate people is part of a balanced lifestyle—and will even improve your digestion! Sharing meals with friends and family is a fantastic way to connect, especially when the conversation is joyful and supportive. Dishes from Part II that are meant to be shared— like Jackfruit Tacos (page 137) and Loaded Baked Sweet Potatoes (page 123)—or the Lunar Ritual recipes (pages 179–193) in Part III can also be opportunities to turn meals into memories.

Connection can also happen on an internal or individual level. If you live alone or just need some time to recharge solo, the Self-Love Self-Massage (page 215) is a beautiful ritual to reconnect to your physical body and feel with your own hands the stability and softness of your shape. Preparing your favorite meal and enjoying it in solitude, perhaps with a calming scented candle or oil diffuser and in the presence of herbal accoutrements, can forge a deep connection between body, mind, and spirit by feeding all three at once. Spending time outdoors is another way to foster connection at the macro-level, and feed your mind with *sattva* (page 154).

SPIRITUALITY

Everyone has a different interpretation of spirituality, and no matter what religion or faith practice you belong to (or don't), you can find ways to connect to the essence of a higher power that unites all beings. Start your day with a few moments of quiet reflection; the time just before dawn, when the light, trees, and animals are suffused with an ethereal calm, is the perfect time to connect to the divine around and inside you. This can look like formal meditation, breathwork, journaling, reading (spiritual texts, poems, but not emails or the news!), spending time outdoors in the elements, walking slowly, or sitting. You might situate your mindfulness practice near your Wellness Altar (see page 201), with a bowl of water containing fresh flowers or herbs to connect you to the beauty and abundance of nature.

FURTHER STUDY

The study of herbs is lifelong and ever-evolving. Here are some of our favorite references for detailed explanations of the medicinal and spiritual aspects of herbs and plant medicine. Before beginning a more specific herbal protocol, please consult with your healthcare provider or holistic practitioner.

+ *Ayurvedic Healing: A Comprehensive Guide*, by David Frawley, Lotus Press, 2001

+ *Balance Your Hormones, Balance Your Life: Achieving Optimal Health and Wellness Through Ayurveda, Chinese Medicine, and Western Science*, by Dr. Claudia Welch, Da Capo Press, 2011

+ *Braiding Sweetgrass: Indigenous Wisdom, Scientific Knowledge, and the Teachings of Plants*, by Robin Wall Kimmerer, Milkweed Editions, 2015

+ *The China Study: The Most Comprehensive Study of Nutrition Ever Conducted and the Startling Implications for Diet, Weight Loss, and Long-Term Health*, by Thomas Campbell and T. Colin Campbell, BenBella Books, 2006

+ *Healing Wise*, by Susan Weed, Ash Tree Publishing, 2003

+ *How Not to Die: Discover the Foods Scientifically Proven to Prevent and Reverse Disease*, by Michael Greger, Flatiron Books, 2015

+ *If Women Rose Rooted: A Life-Changing Journey to Authenticity and Belonging*, by Sharon Blackie, September Publishing, 2019

+ *Medical Herbalism: The Science Principles and Practices of Herbal Medicine*, by David Hoffmann, Healing Arts Press, 2003

+ *Prakriti: Your Ayurvedic Constitution*, by Robert Svoboda, Lotus Press, 1998

+ *The Secret Therapy of Trees: Harness the Healing Energy of Forest Bathing and Natural Landscapes*, by Marco Mencagli and Marco Nieri, Rodale, 2019

+ *The Yoga of Herbs: An Ayurvedic Guide to Herbal Medicine*, by David Frawley and Vasant Lad, Lotus Press, 1986

+ www.americanherbalistsguild.com

+ www.greencomfortherbschool.com

+ www.theherbalacademy.com

+ www.thenaturopathicherbalist.com

+ www.unitedplantsavers.org

HERBAL SUPPLIERS

Treating food as medicine means that your ingredients need to be top-quality and responsibly sourced. Below are our favorite herbal suppliers, who abide by stringent agricultural and labor guidelines to ensure that what you're consuming benefits both you and those who brought it to you. Specific products listed here are based on stock at the time of publication and may be subject to change.

ANIMA MUNDI APOTHECARY

www.animamundiherbals.com

+ Collagen booster
+ Rose powder
+ Reishi powder
+ Mucuna

ANITA'S

www.anitas.com

+ Coconut yogurt

BANYAN BOTANICALS

www.banyanabotanicals.com

FOUR SIGMATIC

www.foursigmatic.com

+ Mushroom blend mix (Defend)
+ Adaptogen blend mix (Chill)

KING ARTHUR FLOUR BLEND

shop.kingarthurflour.com

+ King Arthur's gluten-free measure-for-measure flour is our preferred blend for gluten-free baking, as it makes the best and most authentic substitute for all-purpose flour without graininess or excessive additives.

MAIN COAST SEA VEGETABLES

www.seaveg.com

+ Seaweed (nori, kombu, etc.)

MIYOKO'S CREAMERY

www.miyokos.com

+ Vegan dairy products, including butter and cheese substitutes

MOUNTAIN ROSE HERBS

www.mountainroseherbs.com

NATURE'S CHARM

www.naturescharmveganproducts.com

+ Coconut cream

NAVITAS ORGANICS

www.navitas.com

NUTREX HAWAII

www.nutrex-hawaii.com

+ Spirulina

ACKNOWLEDGMENTS

Food brings people together—that's something we knew going into this book. What we didn't realize, though, was how much people would bring a sense of magic, love, and true nourishment to the food we prepared for the collection of recipes you're holding in your hands. We want to say thank you to all of the people who were part of this journey:

To the generations of healers, teachers, and wise women (and men) who befriended the Earth, learned her secrets, and passed them down through the holistic lineages of herbalism, Ayurveda, yoga, and more.

To our book publishing team, who shared our beliefs in the power of plant healing and helped bring our vision to you—our agent, Marilyn Allen, who saw the future of our mission; our editor, Anja Schmidt, who helped shape our words and advocated for them to be read; her assistant, Samantha Lubash, whose patience and organization ushered these pages through the ether into their current, beautiful form; Matthew Ryan and Patrick Sullivan, whose eyes for composition and artistry brought the aesthetics of this book to a new level; Annie Craig, Laura Jarrett, and Allison Har-zvi in the production department, and copyeditor Ivy McFadden, whose behind-the-scenes wizardry and enviable patience for detail ensured our words were clear, consistent, and accurate; Laura Flavin, Lauren Ollerhead, and Molly Pieper, whose efforts in marketing and publicity made it possible for us to reach you; and Theresa DiMasi, publisher of Tiller, whose leadership and support of creators like us is what keeps us connected in even the most trying times through the education and storytelling that only books can offer.

To our recipe testers—your feedback, advice, and willingness to experiment with our works-in-progress made this book simpler and tastier.

And, most of all, to you, our reader—we hope this book inspires you to see yourself and your health in a new way. We want you to know you are a beautiful, miraculous being, even if you make none of the recipes (though we sure hope you give them a try!). By choosing to prioritize your own well-being through food and self-care, you are contributing to the revolution of healing that is slowly restoring our society and planet to a state of compassion, balance, and wholeness. We, and the universe, thank you for using your energy for that greater good.

—ABBEY & JENNIFER

This work is a culmination of the two roots that shaped my foundation: nature and books. My connection to the earth was born in the forests, brambles, and dirt where I spent my childhood, often with a storybook and a vision for the world playing in my mind. I owe the cultivation of those loves to my mom, who knew what I needed to thrive.

To my parents and sisters—Mom, thank you for showing me how to create, and for instilling in me a fondness for plants. Dad, thank you for always checking in and for your words of encouragement. Ginger, thank you for continually believing in my vision and ideas, and for your unwavering support. Holly, thank you for being an example in grit. Dianne and Tim, thank you for assisting and sharing in the experience of creating this book. Stephanie, thank you for being my everlasting cheerleader and for seeing me. Lindsay, thank you for your insight into the divinity of women.

To my other mothers and sisters—Molly and Katie, thank you for our deeply rooted friendship and sisterhood. Your sustained faith in me through the ebbs and flows of life has always been an anchor, and you both inspire me to show up and make the world better. Mel, thank you for being an original wise woman in my orbit, and for showing me the power of women. Teresa, thank you for teaching the tradition of herbalism and for sharing your healing gifts with me. Charity, thank you for helping me learn about the foundations of health and nutrition and what it means to live well, in all of its forms. Thank you to Rachel, Kim, Chandice, Bekka, and Lisa who reminded me where to find alignment, especially during the creation of this book. And to all of my other family, friends, and mentors whose influence went into this work.

To The Butter Half community—this book would not exist without your support and readership. Thank you for being loyal virtual friends and for joining me in the journey of what it means to root and nourish.

To my kitchen witch sister, Jennifer—thank you for your insight, guidance, and ability to craft our magic into something beautiful.

And finally, to my boys—Matt, Luke, Wes, and Graham—thank you for being taste testers, honest feedback givers, photography assistants, happy helpers, and my emotional support team. Most importantly, thank you for believing in me, and helping me unearth the wise woman who has always dwelled within. I love you.

—ABBEY

Nothing about this book was "supposed" to happen. And yet, here we are, and I am grateful to the twists and turns of fate that have allowed me to share these forms of nourishment with you.

I come from a family of eaters, and while I have not always been a lover of food that part of my DNA resurfaced once I discovered the beauty of cooking and eating from the bounty of our home—the earth. But there was first *my* home, and the people who have built and sustained it. Through all of my ups and downs, my mother and father provided the best nourishment I could have ever imagined—you made sure we always had more than enough food (and only the absolute best-quality produce; no wilty parsley in our kitchen!), and taught me how to prepare it and enjoy it. Most of all, you loved me and called me back home whenever I got lost.

Samantha, you're more than a sister—my forever sidekick, style icon, and rock, you help me realize how much more there is to taste in life.

Thanks to all my extended family—your appetite for trying my vegan recipes and surprise when they were good (and not-so-good) are constant sources of encouragement and entertainment.

And to Katie, Lisa A., Amanda, Lisa W., Brittany, Sierra, Sarah, and Liz—my friends, my chosen family, without whom I'd never have had the courage to take the leaps of faith through life that led me to here and now. Special thanks to Brita and Chris, whose indulgence in these recipes throughout the process helped me refine my palate in all the ways.

The sweet to my bitter, my coauthor and fellow herbal witch, Abbey—our friendship was written in the stars, and I'm grateful for the ways you've helped me grow as a writer, cook, and human. Words won't do justice to how much I admire your heart of fire and grace—but roses might.

Without having edited books first, I never would have been able to write one. My publishing mentors and colleagues at Penguin Random House—Robin Desser, Jenny Jackson, Bob Gottlieb, Kathy Hourigan, and the late Sonny Mehta—and The Experiment—Matthew Lore and Peter Burri—gave me the best education in what makes a good story a great and important book. I hope I've made you proud, despite having gone over to the dark side.

At the Kripalu School of Ayurveda, I found a beautiful *sangha* of fellow students of life—Erin, Lauren, the faculty, and all my peers—who have become lifelong friends and partners on this journey toward peace. You gave me earth when I was falling, water when my well ran dry, fire to light up the dark, air to (re)discover my rhythm and sing from my heart, and space to be. I am grateful to have joined the community of nature ambassadors through these precious teachings.

It's hard to know during times of suffering whether lessons will come from it. Through my experiences of illness and loss, I was given the gifts of yoga, mindfulness, self-study, healthy eating, and a sense of purpose and worth. For the people and spirits who presented me with those gifts, cared for me while we tended my body and soul, and helped me realize their roots inside of me, I say thank you.

—JENNIFER

INDEX

Page numbers in *italics* refer to illustrations.

A

açai berries, recipe using, 74, *75*

Adaptogenic Chocolate Chip Cookies, *206*, 207

Adaptogenic Double Chocolate Brownies, 146, *147*

adaptogenic herbs, 26, 106, 107, 109, 146, 164–165

adrenal glands, 26, 30

adrenal tonics, 30, 106, 107, 164–165

allspice, recipes using, 67

Almond Butter
recipe for, 47
recipes using, 74, 96, 168, 169, 197, 200

almond flour, recipes using, 70, 127, 195

almond meal, recipes using, 96, 141

almond mylk
recipe for, 43
recipes using, 43, 109, 115, 186, 207, 209, 217, 218

almonds, recipes using, 43, 47, 140, 148, 173, 174, 218

altars, 201, *202*, 203

alterative herbs, 26, 164–165

Alternate Nostril Breathing, 143

American skullcap, 159

anise, recipes using, 53, 152

anti-inflammatory herbs, 27, 65, 89

antimicrobial herbs, 27, 65

antioxidant herbs, 27, 65, 90

antispasmodic herbs, 27, 65, 164–165

Anytime Digestive Water, 55

aperient herbs, 27, 65

aphrodisiac herbs, 28, 109, 110, 164–165, 197

Apple Oat Smoothie Bowl, 169

apples, recipes using, 90, 169

aquafaba, 148

artichoke hearts, recipe using, 131

asafoetida, 51, 81

ashwagandha
about, 109, 221
herbal action, 26, 27, 28, 29, 30, 65, 107, 164, 214
recipes using, 67, 74, 109, 110, 127, 153, 174, 195, 198, 207, 209, 214

Asian ginseng
herbal action, 26, 28, 29, 30, 107, 164
recipes using, 109, 204

asparagus, recipe using, 132

astringent herbs, 28, 65, 164–165

Avocado Dip, 191

Avocado Sauerkraut Toast, 66

Avocado Womb Bowl, *178*, 179

avocadoes, recipes using, 66, 115, 137, 145, 179, 191

Ayurveda, 13, 20, 63, 77, 81, 93, 98, 105, 110, 140, 162, 163, 172, 176, 195, 201, 214, 215, 217

Ayurvedic CCF Tea, 82, 98

Ayurvedic psychology, 154

B

Baked Apples with Whipped Coconut Cream, 90, *91*

baked items
Adaptogenic Chocolate Chip Cookies, *206*, 207
Adaptogenic Double Chocolate Brownies, 146, *147*
Chocolate Almond Butter Oat Bars, 96
Essential Banana Bread Muffins, 70, *71*
Happy Lemon Bars, 148
Savory Sage and Flower Tea Biscuits, 141
Sourdough for the Soul, 130

Balanced Beauty Bowl with Schisandra, *166*, 167

balsamic vinegar, 56

Banana Bread Muffins, 70, *71*

bananas, recipes using, 70, 109, 116, 167, 168, 199

basil
form used, 24
herbal action, 27, 28, 65
recipes using, 85, 122, 124, 128–129

basmati rice, recipes using, 76, 77, 81

beans, 51
recipes using, 51, 122, 123, 136, 184

beets
herbal action, 186
recipes using, 86, 184, 186

Belly Yoga, 79

berries
herbal action, 167
recipes using, 74, 93, 110, 120, 167, 210

Berry Probiotic Açai Bowl, 74, *75*

beverages. *See* teas and drinks; teas and drinks recipes

"biophilia," 35

bitter herbs, 28, 65

bitters, 59

black pepper
form used, 24
herbal action, 27, 28, 65
with turmeric, 209

Blackie, Sharon, 20
Bliss Bites, 195, *196*, 197–200
blueberries, recipes using, 110, 120
Blueberry, Rose and Walnut Granola, 110, *111*
breakfast, 220
    recipes for female reproductive health, 167–175
    recipes for good digestion, 66–75
    recipes for mental health, 109–111, 113–117
breakfast recipes
    Apple Oat Smoothie Bowl, 169
    Avocado Sauerkraut Toast, 66
    Balanced Beauty Bowl with Schisandra, *166*, 167
    Berry Probiotic Açaí Bowl, 74, *75*
    Blueberry, Rose and Walnut Granola, 110, *111*
    Chamomile Moong Dal Porridge, 73
    Cherry Vanilla Oats, 114
    Essential Banana Bread Muffins, 70, *71*
    Grain-free Seed Granola—Four Ways, 170, *171*, 172–174
    Mighty Miso Mushroom, 115
    Morning-of Oats, 113–115
    Nuts for Nuts Oats, 114
    Peanut Butter and Elderberry (PBE), 113
    PMS Smoothie, 168
    Scrambled Plants, 115
    smoothies, 74, 109
    Spirulina Bliss Smoothie, *108*, 109
    Vanilla Bean Sweet Potato Banana Pancakes, 116, *117*
    Weekday Chia Seed Puddings, 67–68, *68*
breathing techniques, 118, 143
broccoli, recipes using, 89, 131, 188

brownies, 146
Brussel sprouts, recipes using, 189, 191
buckwheat groats, recipes using, 172, 174, 175

C

cabbage, recipes using, 80, 89
cacao, 101, 164, 197, 198, 214
cacao powder, recipes using, 67, 101, 106, 140, 145, 146, 153, 168, 174, 198, 204, 214
calendula
    herbal action, 26, 27, 29, 30, 65, 164
    recipe using, 99
Calming Vanilla and Oats Chia Seed Pudding, 67–68
cardamom
    form used, 24, 28
    herbal action, 28, 65
    recipes using, 55, 67, 73, 81–82, *83*, 93, 114, 140, 142, 152, 198, 218
carminative herbs, 28, 65, 89
Cashew Cream
    recipe for, 48
    recipes using, 78, 123, 127, 137, 141, 142, 145
cashews, recipes using, 43, 48, 77–78, 131, 175
Cauliflower Pizza with Cashew Cream, Fennel, Arugula, and Honey, *126*, 127
cauliflower rice, 119
cayenne
    form used, 28
    herbal action, 27, 65
    recipes using, 93, 106, 131, 153, 175, 180, 186, 209
Cayenne Cacao, 106
Cayenne Cacao with Tahini, 153, 177
celery root, recipe using, 136
Chai Brown Rice Pudding with Mucuna, 142
chai recipes, 67–68, 142, 152

Chai This Chia Seed Pudding, 67–68
chamomile
    herbal action, 27, 28, 29, 30, 65, 107, 213
    recipes using, 58, 73, 99, 148, 157
Chamomile Moong Dal Porridge, 73
Chamomile Syrup, 148
chard, recipes using, 115, 136
chasteberry, herbal action, 168
cherries, recipes using, 114, 149
Cherry Vanilla Oats, 114
chia seeds
    herbal action, 29, 65
    recipes using, 67–68, 74, 109, 110, 115, 167, 168, 172, 173
chickpea flour, recipe using, 141
chickpeas, recipes using, 51, 86, 148, 180, 197
chicory root, herbal action, 27, 28, 29, 30, 65, 101
Chicory Root Cacao, *100*, 101, 177
chili, 122, 123, 137
Chinese skullcap, 159
chocolate, recipes using, 96, 146, 197, 200, 207, 208
Chocolate Almond Butter Oat Bars, 96
Chunky Fennel, Beet and Chickpea Salsa, 86, *87*
cilantro
    form used, 24
    herbal action, 26, 27, 28, 29, 65, 164
    recipes using, 78, 81–82, 84, 119, 123, 137
cinnamon
    form used, 24
    herbal action, 27, 28, 65, 164
    recipes using, 48, 53, 54, 67, 70, 81–82, *83*, 90, 96, 110, 114, 115, 152, 153, 168, 169, 174, 175, 188, 189, 191, 198, 200, 209, 214, 218

circadian rhythm, 34
citrus fruit, recipes using, 132, 148, 150
Cleansing Spring Water, 54
cloves
    form used, 24
    herbal action, 27, 28, 65
    recipes using, 53, 55, 80, 90, 124, 136, 141, 152, 180, 189, 191, 193–194
coconut, recipes using, 49, 50, 55, 73, 77–78, 80, 85, 110, 114, 123, 128–129, 131, 140, 145, 167, 172, 195, 197, 199, 200, 204
coconut aminos, 124
coconut cream, 49, 90, 145, 148
Coconut Fennel Cashew Curry, 77–78
coconut milk
    about, 43, 164
    recipe for, 43
    recipes using, 67, 78, 142, 204, 214
coconut mylk, 43, 49, 152
coconut sugar, 146, 148, 207
coconut yogurt, 67–68, 74, 90
coffee, 101
congee, 76
connection, as pillar of health, 35, 222
conventional medicine, 14, 106
Cookie Dough Bites, 197
cooking oil, herbal, 58
Cooling Summer Water, 55
coriander, recipes using, 55, 77, 81–82, 83, 98, 132, 173
corn, recipes using, 123
Corpse Pose (yoga), 158
corpus luteum, 174
cortisol, 105
cravings, 16, 17, 33
Creamy Broccoli Soup, 188
Creamy Chai Latte, 152
Crunchy Seaweed Wrap, 182–183
cumin
    form used, 24
    herbal action, 27, 28, 29, 65, 164

recipes using, 55, 77, 81–82, 89, 98, 137, 175, 179, 180, 184, 186
Curate Your Own Wellness Altar, 201, 202, 203
curcumin, 26, 209
curries, 77–78
curry paste, recipes using, 67
Cycle Support Teas, 210, 211

D

daily rituals, 220–222
dandelion greens, 85
dandelion root
    form used, 24
    herbal action, 26, 28, 29, 30, 65
    recipes using, 59
Dark Chocolate Fig Oatmeal Bites, 197
date juice, 48, 182
date syrup, 48, 101
dates, recipes using, 43, 48, 140, 145, 168, 195, 198, 200, 218
Deep Hydration Water, 55
demulcent herbs, 29, 65
deserts. See sweets recipes
digestion
    about, 15, 62–64, 79, 104
    of beans, 51
    bitters for, 59
    constipation, preventing, 79, 97
    good digestion, 62–63
    herbs for, 29, 63, 65, 85, 89
    holistic tradition, 62
    integrative digestion, 63
    microbiome, 64, 66, 74, 86
    peristalsis, 79
    recipes for
        breakfast, 66–75
        digestive tonics, 30
        main dishes, 76–78, 80–93
        sweets, 96
        teas and drinks, 54–55, 96–101

Rule of Threes for Rooted Digestion, 72, 140, 220
    tonics, 30, 65
    yoga for, 79
digestive tonics, 30, 65
dill, recipes using, 132, 179
dips, 131, 191
Double Chocolate Bliss Bites, 200
Double Chocolate Cacao Chia Seed Pudding, 67–68
dressings and sauces, 89, 124, 132
dulse, recipe using, 188

E

eating
    best times for, 72
    daily rituals, 220
    Gratitude Reflection, 112
    mindful eating, 63
    monodiet, 78, 82
    mood and, 141
    Rule of Threes for Rooted Digestion, 72, 140, 220
    schedule for, 220
    seasonal eating, 94–95
    See also food; meals
edible flowers, 141
egg, plant-based, 180
elderberry
    herbal action, 26, 27, 28, 65, 164
    recipes using, 53, 67, 93, 113
Elderberry Syrup
    recipe for, 52, 53
    recipes using, 67, 93, 110, 115
emmenagogue herbs, 29, 164–165
Energizing Sun Salutations, 118, 177
enteric nervous system, 15–16
Essential Banana Bread Muffins, 70, 71
estrogen, 172
eustress, 105
exercise, 34, 221–222

F

fall season, suggested foods, spices, and herbs for, 95
female reproductive health
  about, 16, 162–164
  fertilization, 174
  foods for, 16, 188
  herbs for, 29, 56, 164–165, 217
  hormones, 162–163, 168, 172, 174
  lunar cycles and rituals, 176–177
  menstrual cycle, 168, 170, 172, 174, 177, 188, 217
  ovulation, 172, 174, 177
  recipes for
    breakfast, 167–175
    main dishes, 179–184, 186–194
    sweets, 195–200, 204–208
    teas and drinks, 209–214, 217–218
  uterine tonics, 30, 164–165
  yarrow for, 56
feminine energy, 19
fennel
  form used, 24
  herbal action, 27, 28, 29, 65, 164
  recipes using, 55, 77–78, 81–82, 83, 86, 93, 98, 127, 172, 173, 175
fenugreek
  herbal action, 27, 28, 29, 30, 164, 183, 189
  recipes using, 54, 189, 191
  sprouting seeds, 183
fermented and cultured foods, 64
figs, recipes using, 93, 197, 198
flax meal
  preparing, 70
  recipes using, 96, 109, 110, 115, 127, 140, 141, 146, 172–175

flaxseed
  flax meal from, 70
  form used, 25
  herbal action, 27, 29, 65, 164, 170, 172
follicular phase (menstrual cycle), 172, 188, 210
food cravings. See cravings
foods
  about, 33, 66, 95, 110
  daily rituals, 220
  defined, 14–15
  fermented and cultured, 64
  Gratitude Reflection, 112
  as medicine, 14
  for phases of menstrual cycle, 177
  seasonal eating, 94–95
  stress around, 105
  See also digestion; eating; meals
fudge, 204
full moon rituals, 177

G

Garden Goddess Tonic, 212, 213
garlic
  form used, 24
  herbal action, 27, 28, 65
  recipes using, 48, 85, 86, 89, 127, 131, 137, 186
Gentle Yoga for Relaxation, 158
ginger
  form used, 24
  herbal action, 28, 65, 164
  pickled ginger, 182
  recipes using, 54, 55, 67, 73, 76–78, 80–82, 89, 93, 110, 115, 119, 140, 142, 152, 169, 174, 182, 189, 191, 195, 204, 209, 218
ginseng
  Asian ginseng, 26, 28, 29, 30, 107
  herbal action, 26, 28, 29, 30, 107, 164

Indian ginseng, 109
Peruvian ginseng, 110
recipes using, 109, 119, 204
Ginseng Cilantro Lime Cauliflower Rice, 119
gluten, avoiding, 17
Goddess Pose (yoga), 177
goji berries, recipes using, 110
Golden Cream of Beet Soup, 186, 187
Grain-free Seed Granola—Four Ways, 170, 171, 172–174, 177
granola, 110, 169, 170, 171, 172–174, 177
Grounding and Connecting to Plant Energy, 134, 135, 177

H

Happy Lemon Bars, 148
health
  daily rituals, 220–222
  five pillars of, 33–35, 220–222
  illness, 104
  immune system, 30, 53, 107
  medical care, 106, 163
  self-inquiry questions, 33–35
Healthy Pantry recipes
  Almond Butter, 47
  Cashew Cream, 48
  Dried Beans, 51
  Elderberry Syrup, 52, 53
  Herbal Balsamic Vinegar, 56, 57, 120
  Herbal Cooking Oil, 58
  Herbal Vinegar Bitters, 59
  Herbal Waters, 54–55
  Nuts and Seed Butters, 45–47
  Plant Mylks, 43
  Plant Parmesan, 50
  Pumpkin Seed Butter, 45, 46
  Soaked Dates, 48

Healthy Pantry recipes (*cont.*)
    Tahini, 45, 47
    Umami Spice Blend, 50
    Vanilla Extract, 44
    Whipped Coconut Cream
      with Marshmallow Root,
      49
Heartwarming Vegan Chili,
    122, 123
hemp seeds, recipes using,
    50, 74, 109, 167
hepatic herbs, 29, 65
herbal actions
    adaptogens, 26, 106, 107,
      109, 146, 164–165
    alterative, 26, 164–165
    anti-inflammatory, 27, 65,
      89
    antimicrobial, 27, 65
    antioxidant, 27, 65, 90
    antispasmodic, 27, 65,
      164–165
    aperient, 27, 65
    aphrodisiac, 28, 109, 110,
      164–165, 197
    astringent, 28, 65, 164–165
    bitter, 28, 65
    carminative, 28, 65, 89
    demulcent, 29, 65
    emmenagogue, 29,
      164–165
    hepatic, 29, 65
    laxative, 29, 65
    mood-enhancing, 110
    nervine relaxants, 29, 106,
      107, 157
    phytoestrogenic, 29,
      164–165
    sedative, 29, 106, 107
    tonics, 30, 106, 107,
      164–165, 221
    vulnerary, 30, 65
Herbal Balsamic Vinegar
    recipe for, 56, *57*
    recipes using, 120, 189, 191
Herbal Cooking Oil
    recipe for, 58
    recipes using, 120, 137,
      179, 180
Herbal Lullaby Tea, 159
herbal medicine, 14

Herbal Vinegar Bitters, 59,
    149
Herbal Waters, 54–55
herbalism, 18–19
herbs
    about, 14, 162
    for digestion, 29, 63, 65,
      85, 89
    for female reproductive
      health, 29, 56, 164–165
    form used, 24–25
    herbal actions, 26–30,
      63, 65, 85, 89, 106, 107,
      164–165
    herbal pantry, 40–59
    for mental health, 106, 107
    resources for study, 223
    suppliers of, 224
    use of small quantities, 18
    using, 23, 106
hibiscus
    herbal action, 28, 29, 164
    recipes using, 210, 217
Himalayan sea salt, 72
hing
    form used, 24, 51
    herbal action, 27, 28, 65
    recipes using, 51, 81–82,
      83
holistic healing, 13, 14
Holy Basil, 217
honey, 17–18, 98
hormones, 16, 105, 162–163,
    168, 172, 174
    See also female
      reproductive health
hummus, 66, 184

illness, 104
immune system, 30, 53, 107
immune tonics, 30, 107
Indian ginseng, 109
inflammation, reduction of,
    27
infused vinegar, 56
integrative digestion, 63
inulin, 101

Jackfruit Tacos, 137, *138–139*

kale, recipes using, 109, 188
kimchi, recipe using, 80
kitchari, 81–82, *83*
kitchen equipment, 36–37
kombu, recipes using, 51, 76,
    80, 115

lattes, 26, 152, 177, 209
lavender
    form used, 24
    herbal action, 27, 28, 29,
      107, 157, 165
    recipes using, 141, 157
Lavender, Chamomile and
    Rose Tea, *156*, 157
laxative herbs, 29, 65
Leafy Greens Salad with
    Walnuts and Berries, 120,
    121
Left Side Down Posture, 79
lemon balm
    form used, 24
    herbal action, 27, 28, 29,
      107, 150
    recipes using, 137, 150
Lemon Balm Lemonade, 150,
    151
lemon bars, 148
lemon water, 97
lemonade, 150, *151*
lemongrass
    form used, 24
    herbal action, 28, 29, 107,
      165
    recipes using, 124, 137
Lemongrass Spring Rolls
    with Tempeh, 124, *125*,
    182

lentils, 51
    recipes using, 122, 179, 186
licorice root
    form used, 24
    herbal action, 26, 27, 29,
        30, 65, 99, 107, 165, 204
    recipes using, 89, 99, 159,
        168, 204, 209, 217
liver
    elderberry syrup for, 93
    hepatic herbs, 29, 65
    tonics, 30
Loaded Baked Sweet
    Potatoes, 123
lunar cycles and rituals,
    176–177
lunch, 220
luteal phase (menstrual
    cycle), 174, 210

M

maca
    form used, 110
    herbal action, 28, 29, 107,
        110, 165
    recipes using, 110, 114, 115,
        167, 172, 173, 197, 199,
        207, 214
main dish recipes
    Avocado Womb Bowl, *178*,
        179
    Cauliflower Pizza with
        Cashew Cream, Fennel,
        Arugula, and Honey,
        126, 127
    Chunky Fennel, Beet and
        Chickpea Salsa, 86, *87*
    Coconut Fennel Cashew
        Curry, 77–78
    Creamy Broccoli Soup, 188
    Crunchy Seaweed Wrap,
        182–183
    Ginseng Cilantro Lime
        Cauliflower Rice, 119
    Golden Cream of Beet
        Soup, 186, *187*
    Heartwarming Vegan Chili,
        122, 123

Jackfruit Tacos, 137,
    138–139
Leafy Greens Salad with
    Walnuts and Berries,
    120, *121*
Lemongrass Spring Rolls
    with Tempeh, 124, *125*
Loaded Baked Sweet
    Potatoes, 123
Mushroom Risotto with
    Spinach, Peas and
    Nettles, *192*, 193–194
Probiotic Quinoa Cabbage
    Stir-Fry, 80
Restorative Kitchari,
    81–82, *83*
Roasted Brussel Sprouts,
    Sweet Potato and
    Tempeh Bowl with
    Fenugreek Dressing,
    189, *190*, 191
Shakshuka with Plant-
    Based Egg, 180, *181*
Slow and Simple Congee,
    76
Spaghetti Squash Boats
    with Basil and Oregano,
    128–129
Spinach Artichoke Cashew
    Dip, 131
Thai Peanut Stir-Fry with
    Tofu, *88*, 89
Warm Winter Citrus Salad,
    132, *133*
White Bean Beet Hummus,
    184
White Bean Celery Root
    Soup with Thyme and
    Rosemary, 136
Wild Dandelion and Mint
    Pesto, *84*, 85
main dishes
    about, 220, 221
    recipes for female
        reproductive health,
        179–184, 186–194
    recipes for good digestion,
        76–78, 80–93
    recipes for mental health,
        119–129, 131–132,
        136–140

male reproductive system,
    ashwagandha for, 109
maple syrup, recipes using,
    148, 153, 172, 174, 204, 209
marshmallow root
    herbal action, 29, 65
    recipes using, 49
masculine energy, 19
massage oils, 215
Matcha Bites, 195
meals
    best times for, 72
    daily rituals, 220
    Rule of Threes for Rooted
        Digestion, 72, 140, 220
    schedule for, 220
    timing of, 220–221
    See also eating; food
medical care, 106, 163
menstrual cycle
    about, 168, 170, 177, 188,
        217
    follicular phase, 172, 188,
        210
    lunar cycles and rituals,
        177
    luteal phase, 174, 210
mental health
    about, 15–16, 104–106
    Ayurvedic psychology, 154
    foods for, 16
    herbs for, 106, 107
    recipes for
        breakfast, 109–111,
            113–117
        main dishes, 119–129,
            131–132 136–140
        sweets, 140–142,
            144–148
        teas and drinks,
            149–153, 157, 159
mental illness, 105
microbiome, 64, 66, 74, 86
Mighty Miso Mushroom, 115
Milk Thistle and Nettle Tea,
    177, 210
milky oats, 142
mindful eating, 63
mineral salt, 82
mint, recipes using, 55, 85,
    93, 120, 145

Mint Cacao Avocado Pudding, *144*, 145
miso, recipes using, 80, 89, 115, 119, 131, 132, 182
Miso-Tahini Spread, 182
moderation, 18
monodiet, 78, 82
mood, eating and, 141
mood-enhancing herbs, 110
moon, lunar cycles and rituals for women, 176–177
moon bathing, 177
Moon Glow Bites, 199
moong dal, recipes using, 73, 81–82, *83*
Morning-of Oats, 113–115
movement, as pillar of health, 34, 221–222
mucuna
    herbal action, 28, 29, 30, 107, 110, 165
    recipes using, 110, 140, 153
mung beans, recipes using, 73, 81–82, *83*
mushroom powder, recipe using, 146
Mushroom Risotto with Spinach, Peas and Nettles, *192*, 193–194
mushrooms, recipes using, 80, 115, 193–194
mustard seeds, recipe using, 136

N

nervous system
    nervine relaxants, 29, 106, 107, 157
    sedative herbs, 29, 106, 107
    tonics for, 30, 106, 107
nettles
    herbal action, 27, 29, 30, 165
    recipes using, 56, 58, 188, 193–194, 210
new moon rituals, 177

nigella seeds, recipes using, 189, 191
nonndairy cheese substitutes, 50
nori seaweed, 182–183
nutmeg, recipes using, 90, 93, 115, 142, 152, 179
nutrition, as pillar of health, 33
nuts, recipes using, 43, 45–47, 48, 70, 110, 114, 120, 131, 173–175
nuts and seed butters
    recipes for, 45–47
    recipes using, 00, 74, 89, 96, 168, 169, 197
Nuts for Nuts Oats, 114

O

oat mylk, 43, 153
oats, 73, 113, 142
    Apple Oat Smoothie Bowl, 169
    Baked Apples with Whipped Coconut Cream, 90
    Blueberry, Rose and Walnut Granola, 110
    Cherry Vanilla Oats, 114
    Chocolate Almond Butter Oat Bars, 96
    Dark Chocolate Fig Oatmeal Bites, 197
    Essential Banana Bread Muffins, 70
    Happy Lemon Bars, 148
    Matcha Bites, 195
    Mighty Miso Mushroom, 115
    Moon Glow Bites, 199
    Morning-Of Oats, 113–115
    Nuts for Nuts Oats, 114
    Peanut Butter and Elderberry (PBE), 113
    Plant Mylks, 43
    preparing, 113
    Pumpkin Seed Cacao Bites, 198
    Scrambled Plants, 115

Vanilla Bean Sweet Potato Banana Pancakes, 116
    Weekday Chia Seed Pudding, 67–68
oatstraw
    herbal action, 27, 28, 29, 30, 107, 165
    recipes using, 142, 152
oils, 164
ojas, 218, 219
Ojas Mylk, 218
ovulation, 172, 174, 177

P

pancakes, 116
paprika, recipes using, 115, 137, 175, 180, 189, 191
parasympathetic hormones, 163
parmesan cheese, vegan, 50, 85, 123, 128–129, 131, 193–194
parsley
    form used, 25
    herbal action, 28, 65
    recipes using, 123, 132
passionflower
    about, 149
    herbal action, 27, 29, 107
    recipes using, 149, 159
Passionflower Mocktail, 149
peanut butter, recipes using, 89, 113, 204
Peanut Butter and Elderberry (PBE), 113
Peanut Butter Licorice Fudge, 204, *205*
peanut sauce, 89, 124
peas, recipe using, 193–194
peppermint
    form used, 25
    herbal action, 27, 28, 29, 65, 165
    recipes using, 99
Peppermint Licorice Tea, 99
peristalsis, 79
Peruvian ginseng, 110
pesto, 85

phytoestrogenic herbs, 29, 164–165

phytoestrogens, 164, 198

Pickled Ginger, 182

Pillars of Health, 33–35, 220–222

Pink Moon Mylk, 217

pistachios, recipe using, 173

pizza, *126*, 127

Plant-Based Egg, 180

plant energy, *134*, 135, 177

Plant Mylks, 43, 109, 115, 168, 186, 207, 209, 217, 218

Plant Parmesan
    recipe for, 50
    recipes using, 85, 123, 128–129, 131, 193–194

PMS Smoothie, 168

porridges, 73, 76

pranayama, 143

prebiotics, 64, 74, 101

Probiotic Elderberry Chia Seed Pudding, 67–68

Probiotic Quinoa Cabbage Stir-Fry, 80

probiotics
    about, 64, 66, 75
    recipes, 67–68, 74, 80

progesterone, 174

prostaglandins, 27

psyllium
    form used, 25
    herbal action, 27, 29, 65
    recipe using, 67

puddings, 67–68, 142, 145

Pumpkin Seed Butter, 45, 46

Pumpkin Seed Cacao Bites, 198

pumpkin seeds
    herbal action, 29, 164, 170, 172, 198
    recipes using, 45, 46, 140, 170, 172, 173, 198

Q

quinoa, recipes using, 80, 110, 173, 188

raspberry leaf, recipe using, 217

red raspberry leaf
    herbal action, 28, 29, 30, 165
    recipes using, 177, 210
    Red Raspberry Leaf and Hibiscus Tea, 177, 210

reishi
    form used, 25
    herbal action, 26, 27, 30, 65, 107, 165
    recipes using, 50, 67, 89, 90, 168, 180, 207

relaxants, 29

REM sleep, 34

rest, as pillar of health, 34

Restorative Kitchari, 81–82, *83*

rice, recipes using, 76, 77, 81, 89, 142, 193–194

rice pudding, 142

risotto, *192*, 193–194

rituals
    daily rituals, 220–222
    lunar cycles and rituals, 176–177

Roasted Brussel Sprouts, Sweet Potato and Tempeh Bowl with Fenugreek Dressing, 189, *190*, 191

Rooted Living tips, 17
    Alternate Nostril Breathing, 143
    Ayurvedic Psychology, 154
    Belly Yoga, 79
    Curate Your Own Wellness Altar, 201, *202*, 203
    Energizing Sun Salutations, 118
    Gentle Yoga for Relaxation, 158
    Gratitude Reflection, 112
    Grounding and Connecting to Plant Energy, *134*, 135
    Moon Glow: Lunar Cycles and Rituals to Connect to the Divine Feminine, 176–177

Rule of Threes for Rooted Digestion, 72, 140, 220

Seasonal Eating, 94–95

Self-Massage, 177, 215

Sourdough for the Soul, 130

Supported Goddess Pose, 185

Your Ojas is Glowing, 219

rose
    form used, 25, 214
    herbal action, 27, 28, 29, 30, 107, 165, 214
    recipes using, 55, 157, 167, 214, 217

Rose Cacao, 177, 214

rose hips, 214

Rule of Threes for Rooted Digestion, 72, 140, 220

S

sage
    form used, 25
    herbal action, 27, 28, 29
    recipe using, 141

salad dressings. *See* dressings and sauces

salads
    Leafy Greens Salad with Walnuts and Berries, 120, *121*
    Warm Winter Citrus Salad, 132, *133*

salt, 82

sauces and dressings, 89, 124, 132

Sauerkraut, recipe using, 66

Savory Green Goddess Chia Seed Pudding, 67–68

Savory Sage and Flower Tea Biscuits, 141

schisandra
    herbal action, 28, 165
    recipe using, 167

Scrambled Plants, 115

sea salt, 72

seasonal eating, 94–95

seaweed, 182
sedative herbs, 29, 106, 107
seed cycling, 170
seed recipes
 Nuts and Seed Butters,
  45–47
 Super Seed Squares, 140
 See also chia seeds;
  sunflower seeds
seeds, 25, 162, 164
self-massage, 177, 215
serotonin, 15
sesame seeds
 form used, 25
 herbal action, 29, 164, 170,
  174
 recipes using, 45, 47, 80,
  119, 140, 170
Shakshuka with Plant-Based
 Egg, 180, *181*
shatavari
 about, 199, 221
 form used, 25
 herbal action, 28, 165, 199,
  214
 recipes using, 172, 197,
  199, 204, 207, 214
shiitake
 form used, 25
 herbal action, 26, 30, 107,
  165
 recipe using, 207
sitting posture, 79
skullcap
 herbal action, 27, 29, 30,
  107, 159
 recipe using, 159
sleep, as pillar of health, 34,
 221
smoothies, 74, 109, 168, 169
snacks, 96, 220
 See also sweets; sweets
  recipes
Soaked Dates
 recipe for, 48
 recipes using, 140, 145,
  169, 186, 195, 218
social connection, as pillar of
 health, 35, 222
soups, 136, 186, 188
Sourdough for the Soul, 130

Spaghetti Squash Boats
 with Basil and Oregano,
 128–129
Spiced Fig and Berry
 Compote, *92*, 93
Spicy Turmeric Latte, 26, 177,
 209
spinach, recipes using, 109,
 115, 120, 122, 128–129, 131,
 193–194
Spinach Artichoke Cashew
 Dip, 131
spirituality, as pillar of health,
 35, 222
spirulina
 form used, 25
 herbal action, 27, 106, 109
 recipes using, 109
Spirulina Bliss Smoothie, 106,
 108, 109
spring season, suggested
 foods, spices, and herbs
 for, 95
spring rolls, 124, *125*
squats (exercise), 79
stir-fry recipes, 80, *88*, 89
strawberries, recipe using,
 120
stress, 104–105
stress hormones, 26
stress response, 16, 104, 163
summer, suggested foods,
 spices, and herbs for, 95
Sun Salutations, 118
sunflower seeds
 herbal action, 29, 164, 170,
  174
 recipes using, 93, 110, 140,
  170, 174, 175
Super Seed Squares, 140
superfoods, 109, 110, 116, 164
Supported Child's Pose
 (yoga), 158
Supported Fish Pose (yoga),
 158
Supported Goddess Pose
 (yoga), 185
sustainable herbalism, 19
sweet potatoes, recipes
 using, 116, 122, 123, 189,
 191

sweets
 recipe for good digestion,
  96
 recipes for female
  reproductive health,
  195–200, 204–208
 recipes for mental health,
  140–142, 144–148
 as snacks, 96, 220
sweets recipes
 Adaptogenic Chocolate
  Chip Cookies, *206*, 207
 Adaptogenic Double
  Chocolate Brownies,
  146, *147*
 Baked Apples with
  Whipped Coconut
  Cream, 90, *91*
 Bliss Bites, 195, *196*,
  197–200
 breakfast recipe, 67–68,
  68
 Chai Brown Rice Pudding
  with Mucuna, 142
 Chocolate Almond Butter
  Oat Bars, 96
 Cookie Dough Bites,
  197
 Dark Chocolate Fig
  Oatmeal Bites, 197
 Double Chocolate Bliss
  Bites, 200
 Happy Lemon Bars,
  148
 Matcha Bites, 195
 Mint Cacao Avocado
  Pudding, *144*, 145
 Moon Glow Bites, 199
 Peanut Butter Licorice
  Fudge, 204, *205*
 Pumpkin Seed Cacao
  Bites, 198
 recipes for good digestion,
  96
 Savory Sage and Flower
  Tea Biscuits, 141
 Spiced Fig and Berry
  Compote, *92*, 93
 Super Seed Squares,
  140
 Tahini Truffles, 208

Weekday Chia Seed
    Puddings, 67–68, *68*
syrups, 48, 53, 101, 148

T

tahini, 45
    recipe for, 47
    recipes using, 114, 115,
        131, 132, 153, 174, 175,
        182, 184, 188, 199, 208
Tahini Miso Dressing, 132
Tahini Truffles, 208
tamari, recipes using, 119,
    182, 189, 191
teas and drinks, 221
    equipment for preparing
        tea, 37
    honey in hot drinks, 18
    preparing herbal tea
        blends, 210
    recipes for female
        reproductive health,
        209–214, 217–218
    recipes for good digestion,
        54–55, 96–101
    recipes for mental health,
        149–153, 157, 159
teas and drinks recipes
    Ayurvedic CCF Tea, 82, 98
    Cayenne Cacao with Tahini,
        153
    Chicory Root Cacao, *100*,
        101
    Cooked Water with Lemon,
        97
    Creamy Chai Latte, 152
    Cycle Support Teas, 210,
        211
    Garden Goddess Tonic,
        212, 213
    Herbal Lullaby Tea, 159
    Lavender, Chamomile and
        Rose Tea, *156*, 157
    Lemon Balm Lemonade,
        150, *151*
    Milk Thistle and Nettle
        Tea, 210
    Ojas Mylk, 218

Passionflower Mocktail,
    149
Peppermint Licorice Tea,
    99
Pink Moon Mylk, 217
Red Raspberry Leaf and
    Hibiscus Tea, 210
Rose Cacao, 177, 214
Spicy Turmeric Latte, 209
Spirulina Bliss Smoothie,
    108, 109
tempeh, recipes using, 124,
    189, 191
Thai Peanut Stir-Fry with
    Tofu, *88*, 89
thyme
    form used, 25
    herbal action, 28, 56, 165
    recipes using, 50, 56, 175,
        193–194
tofu
    how to use, 78
    recipes using, 77–78, 80,
        89, 128–129
tonics, 30, 106, 107, 109,
    164–165, 213, 221
tulsi
    about, 149, 217
    herbal action, 26, 27, 28,
        29, 30, 107, 165, 217
    recipes using, 149, 159,
        217
turmeric
    form used, 25, 209
    herbal action, 26, 27, 28,
        30, 65, 107, 165
    recipes using, 48, 54, 73,
        76, 77, 80, 81–82, 89,
        115, 167, 175, 180, 189,
        191, 209, 218
turnips, recipes using, 136

U

umami, 50, 119
Umami Spice Blend
    recipe for, 50
    recipes using, 115
uterine tonics, 30, 164–165

V

vanilla, 116, 142
Vanilla Bean Sweet Potato
    Banana Pancakes, 116, *117*
Vanilla Extract, 44
vegan cheese, 50
vinegar
    Herbal Balsamic Vinegar,
        56, *57*, 120
    Herbal Vinegar Bitters, 59,
        149
vitex
    herbal action, 165, 168
    recipe using, 168
vulnerary herbs, 30, 65

W

walking, 34, 79
walnuts, recipes using, 70,
    110, 114, 120, 140, 174
Warm Winter Citrus Salad,
    132, *133*
Warming Digestive Water,
    54
water
    Cooked Water with Lemon,
        97
    Herbal Waters, 54–55
watermelon, recipe using,
    120
Weekday Chia Seed Puddings,
    67–68, *68*
wellness altar, 201, *202*, 203
Western herbalism, 13, 20
Western medicine, 14
Whipped Coconut Cream with
    Marshmallow Root
    recipe for, 49
    recipes using, 90, 145
White Bean Beet Hummus,
    184
White Bean Celery Root Soup
    with Thyme and Rosemary,
    136
whole-food plant-based diet,
    63

Wild Dandelion and Mint
    Pesto, *84*, 85
Wind-Relieving Pose (yoga),
    158
winter, suggested foods,
    spices, and herbs for, 95
winter cherry, 109
wound healing, vulnerary
    herbs, 30

Y

yarrow
    herbal action, 27, 28, 29,
        30, 65, 165
    recipes using, 58, 99
yoga, 17, 34, 79, 158, 177,
    185
yogurt. *See* coconut yogurt

ABOUT THE AUTHORS

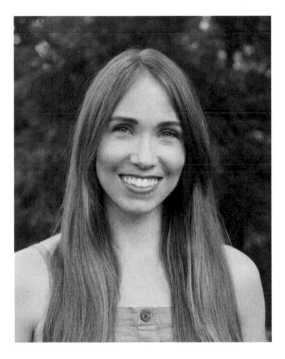

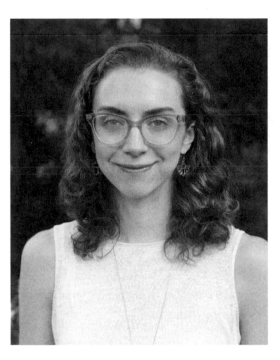

ABBEY RODRIGUEZ is a Certified Holistic Nutritionist, herbalist, and food content creator. Since 2015, she has been developing recipes for women and young families on her food and wellness blog, The Butter Half. She is deeply passionate about the power of plants and nutrition, and teaching others about holistic wellness. She lives in Northern Virginia with her husband and three children.

www.thebutterhalf.com

JENNIFER KURDYLA is an Ayurvedic Health Counselor, yoga teacher, and writer. Plant-based since 2008, she learned to love food by experimenting with vegan and Ayurvedic cooking in her tiny New York kitchens. She lives in Brooklyn.

www.benourished.me

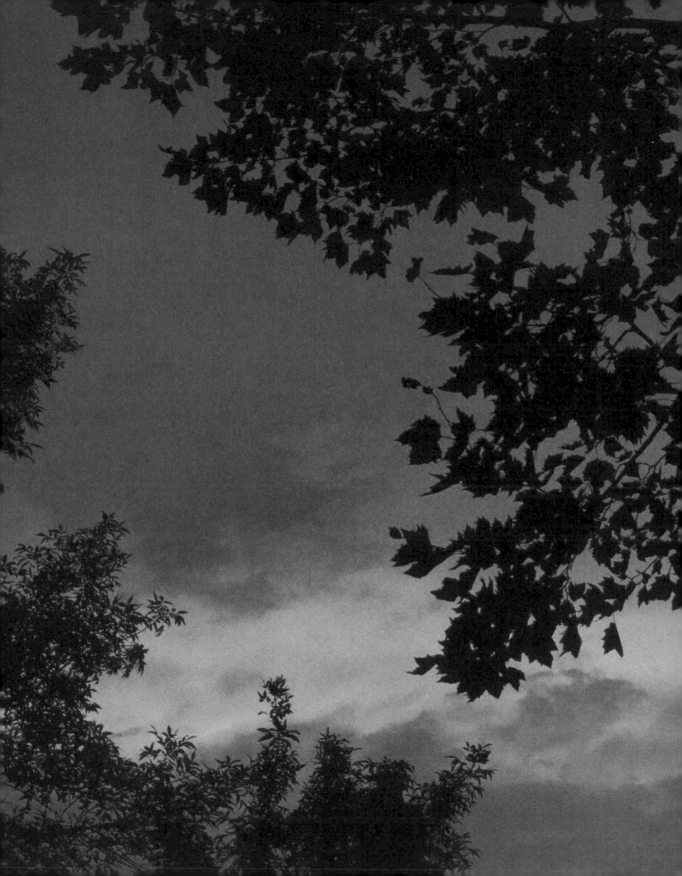